HIV Treatment and Prevention Technologies in International Perspective

Also by Mark Davis
SEX, TECHNOLOGY AND PUBLIC HEALTH

Also by Corinne Squire
CULTURE IN PSYCHOLOGY (*edited*)

DOING NARRATIVE RESEARCH (*co-edited*)

HIV IN SOUTH AFRICA

LINES OF NARRATIVE (*co-edited*)

MORALITY USA (*co-authored*)

PUBLIC EMOTIONS (*co-edited*)

SIGNIFICANT DIFFERENCES: Feminism in Psychology

WOMEN AND HIV: Psychological Perspectives (*edited*)

HIV Treatment and Prevention Technologies in International Perspective

Edited by

Mark Davis
Monash University, Australia

Corinne Squire
University of East London, UK

palgrave
macmillan

First published 2010 by
PALGRAVE MACMILLAN

Palgrave Macmillan in the UK is an imprint of Macmillan Publishers Limited, registered in England, company number 785998, of Houndmills, Basingstoke, Hampshire RG21 6XS.

Palgrave Macmillan in the US is a division of St Martin's Press LLC, 175 Fifth Avenue, New York, NY 10010.

Palgrave Macmillan is the global academic imprint of the above companies and has companies and representatives throughout the world.

Palgrave® and Macmillan® are registered trademarks in the United States, the United Kingdom, Europe and other countries.

ISBN 978–0–230–23819–0 hardback

This book is printed on paper suitable for recycling and made from fully managed and sustained forest sources. Logging, pulping and manufacturing processes are expected to conform to the environmental regulations of the country of origin.

A catalogue record for this book is available from the British Library.

A catalog record for this book is available from the Library of Congress.

10 9 8 7 6 5 4 3 2 1
19 18 17 16 15 14 13 12 11 10

Printed and bound in Great Britain by
CPI Antony Rowe, Chippenham and Eastbourne

Contents

Acknowledgements

This edited collection arises out of a seminar, 'HIV technology and subjectivity: international case studies of HIV treatment and prevention', organised by Mark Davis and Corinne Squire and held on 12 April 2007 at the British Sociological Association (BSA) Annual Conference at the University of East London. The theme of the BSA conference was 'Social connections: identities, technologies, relationships'. Picking up on this theme, the 'HIV technology' seminar reflected on case studies from Africa, Europe and Asia. The chapters in this book are based on presentations at the seminar or on the works of those who were invited but could not attend. We are grateful to the BSA and the conference organisers at the University of East London for supporting the seminar and therefore the opportunity to lay the groundwork for this edited collection. We would also like to thank the anonymous reviewers of the manuscript for their advice.

The cover image appears courtesy the Bambanani Women's Group, Khayelitsha, Cape Town, South Africa. For more information, please see: http://www.memorybox.co.za/index.php?option=com_content&task=view&id=16&Itemid=37

For the book *Long Life ... Positive HIV Stories*, by Jonathan Morgan and the Bambanani Women's Group in collaboration with the Centre for Social Science Research, University of Cape Town, Médecins sans Frontières, and Jane Solomon (2003: Double Storey Press), featuring body maps and autobiographies, please see http://www.doublestorey.com/catalogue/itemdisplay.jsp?item_id=8332

Biographical Notes

Fareed Abdullah headed the Western Cape AIDS programmes from 1996 to 2005. He then moved to the International AIDS Alliance, and in 2008 took on his present duties at the Global Fund to Fight AIDS, Tuberculosis and Malaria as Africa Unit Director. Abdullah has presented and published widely and internationally, particularly in the fields of prevention of mother-to-child HIV transmission treatment, and ART, especially ART scale-up.

Catherine Campbell is Professor of Social Psychology at the London School of Economics where she is Director of the M.Sc. in Health, Community and Development (http://psych.lse.ac.uk/hcd). She is also Adjunct Professor at the University of KwaZulu-Natal. She is a community health psychologist with a particular interest in the link between grass roots community participation and health in marginalised communities – particularly in the context of the HIV/AIDS epidemic – and how the best efforts of communities are hampered by lack of wider political will to tackle the epidemic. She has published widely in international journals, and is the author of *Letting them Die: Why HIV/AIDS Prevention Programmes Fail* (2003, James Currey/ Indiana University Press).

Mark Davis is Lecturer in the School of Political and Social Inquiry, Faculty of Arts, Monash University. Mark has worked in public health practice and research in the UK and Australia with reference to blood-borne viruses such as HIV and hepatitis C. This work has included the impact of ART and related biomedical technologies on sexual practice. His research focuses on empirical and theoretical inquiry that furthers a critical public health for HIV and related concerns. In 2009, Mark published *Sex, Technology and Public Health* with Palgrave Macmillan.

Paul Flowers is Professor of Sexual Health Psychology, Department of Psychology, Glasgow Caledonian University. Paul has conducted a wide range of mixed methods psychosocial research in the area of HIV/AIDS. This has ranged from evaluations of major health promotion campaigns to projects concerning the social impacts of HIV treatments in the lives of people with HIV and their carers in London and Glasgow (the latter funded as part of the ESRC Innovative Health Technologies Programme).

He is a trustee of the National AIDS Trust (NAT) and a member of the National Sexual Health and HIV Advisory Committee, Scotland.

Mike Michael is Professor of Sociology of Science and Technology, and Director of the Centre for the Study of Invention and Social Process, at the Sociology Department, Goldsmiths, University of London. His main areas of research include public understanding of science, the relation between everyday life and mundane technology, and biotechnological and biomedical innovation and culture. He is currently developing an interest in the interactions between design and social science disciplines. Recent publications include *Technoscience and Everyday Life* (Open University Press, 2006), and (with Lynda Birke and Arnie Arluke) *The Sacrifice: How Scientific Experiments Transform Animals and People* (Purdue University Press, 2007).

Eric Mykhalovskiy is an associate professor and Canadian Institutes of Health Research New Investigator in the Department of Sociology, York University. His work on HIV/AIDS draws on studies in the social organisation of knowledge perspective and explores shifts in the relationship between HIV prevention and treatment, the criminalisation of HIV transmission/exposure and the relationship between formal discourses of knowledge and 'lay' experiences of health. He is co-author with Lorna Weir of *Global Public Health Vigilance: Creating a World on Alert* (Routledge, 2009) and co-editor with Marsha Rosengarten in 'HIV/AIDS in its third decade: renewed critique in social and cultural analysis', a special issue of *Social Theory and Health* (2009).

Kane Race is a Senior Lecturer in Gender and Cultural Studies at the University of Sydney. He has published widely on the impact of HIV antiretroviral therapy on gay social and sexual cultures, and the subjugated ethics of sexual and drug-using practices in this context. His book *Pleasure Consuming Medicine: The Queer Politics of Drugs* (Duke University Press, 2009) investigates the political significance of drug discourses in neoliberal society, and the possibilities of 'counterpublic health'.

Marsha Rosengarten is a Lecturer and Deputy Director of the Centre for the Study of Invention and Social Process, at the Sociology Department, Goldsmiths, University of London and Adjunct Research Fellow, National Centre in HIV Social Research, University of New South Wales. Her main areas of research include biomedical innovations in science and medicine, HIV, blood, organ and xenotransplantation, drugs and clinical trials. She is the author of *HIV Interventions: Biomedicine and the Traffic in Information and Flesh* (University of Washington Press, 2009).

Corinne Squire is co-director of the Centre for Narrative Research and Professor of Social Sciences at the University of East London. Recent publications include *HIV in South Africa: Talking about the Big Thing* (London: Routledge, 2007) and *Doing Narrative Research* (edited with Molly Andrews and Maria Tamboukou, London: Sage, 2008). Corinne's research interests are in HIV and citizenship, popular culture and subjectivities, and narrative theory and methods.

Lindy Wilbraham is Professor of Psychology at Rhodes University, Grahamstown, South Africa. She teaches within developmental, social and health psychologies, and discursive and narrative approaches to qualitative research. Her research interests circle around critical public health issues, with particular attention to youth, gender/race/class, women, families and parenting, HIV/AIDS, media, embodiment and power.

1
HIV Technologies

Mark Davis and Corinne Squire

HIV technologies, treatment possibility and health governance

This edited collection addresses the governance of the HIV and AIDS pandemic with reference to the social aspects of technology in international contexts. The term 'technology' is used to encompass medical technologies such as HIV treatment, but also other 'technologies' of health care, including psychosocial and social interventions and communications media applied to moderate HIV's impact and to prevent HIV transmission. HIV technologies of the biomedical kind have become a focus in the research and policy literature. Policy frameworks advocate for close attention to the relationship between HIV treatment and prevention (Global HIV Prevention Working Group, 2008: 6; see also Mykhalovskiy, this volume) and an address to 'psychosocial' factors (UNAIDS, 2009b), as well as integration between HIV and other health and social policy initiatives, around for instance TB, drug use, and gender-based violence (UNAIDS, 2009a). Researchers have warned of the need to consider the social and cultural dimensions of biomedical interventions such as male circumcision (Peltzer et al., 2007). This volume contributes to these debates by investigating the social and cultural dimensions of HIV technologies that find expression in different parts of the world.

While much has been written about the HIV pandemic, recent social scientific research is largely directed at description and policy improvement. For some time now, we have lacked a sustained social science engagement with the pandemic that addresses the changing technologies of its governance. We also lack texts that consider HIV technologies globally. From time to time, inspiring research does appear in the literature, some of it produced by the contributors to this collection.

However, we argue that there is still a need to bring together, and reflect on, theoretically informed, innovative research from different parts of the world concerning the current circumstances of the HIV/AIDS pandemic.

HIV/AIDS is now a true pandemic, affecting people in all parts of the world. UNAIDS (2009c) suggests that 33.4 million people are living with HIV worldwide, with generally decreasing numbers of new infections, but increasing prevalence in some areas, particularly eastern Europe and central Asia. Prevalence is also high within particular groups in some regions – for instance, among black people in the US (Centers for Disease Control, 2009) – and new infections among gay men are increasing in western and central Europe and North America (UNAIDS, 2009c). The pandemic is also radically dynamic and uncertain. For example, HIV prevalence in Uganda fell in the 1990s and then stabilised; now, sexual behaviours that carry HIV transmission risk are reported to be rising (UNAIDS, 2009c). Many prevalence estimates are problematic and contested and error-prone, as indicated in India's National AIDS Control Organisation's 2007 halving of its prevalence figures on the basis of expanded surveillance.

One of the key dimensions of the HIV pandemic was the development of HIV treatment in the mid-1990s. Up to that time, we lacked effective antiviral treatment for HIV infection. In the mid-1990s however, combinations of antiviral drug treatments, now most commonly referred to as antiretroviral therapy, or ART, were found to inhibit viral replication, therefore preventing the deterioration of, and in many cases restoring, the immune systems of people with HIV. Such advantageous medical technologies have had multiple effects. In the affluent countries of the developed world, they have changed the apocalyptic character of public discourse regarding HIV and AIDS. Today in the developed world, HIV is often characterised as a chronic and manageable disease. Improved treatment technologies have also changed the shape of developed-world HIV advocacy and activism. Earlier community action projects were predicated on the imperatives of non-discrimination, care provision, education, transmission reduction and treatment advocacy. In the post-treatment situation, community action has come to focus on the politics of treatment rationing, and on short- and long-term difficulties and possibilities involved with ART such as treatment compliance, side effects, drug 'holidays', simplified medication regimes and the development of new lines of ART. New kinds of relationships between people with HIV and medical services have also been fashioned, often governed by a pronounced medicalised rationality and focused on the technological control of the virus in the body of the individual patient. These technologised relations also include negotiated relationships between doctors and 'expert' patients; increasingly long periods of medicated but unmonitored, 'normalised', HIV life; the common parallel use of complementary and alternative medicine; experiences or expectations of ART problems and failure. Because ART reduces viral activity, debate has also focused on ART's impact on the chance of HIV transmission through sexual intercourse, and how people with HIV address this knowledge in their sexual relationships. These aspects of HIV treatment and prevention raise new and urgent questions about how to effectively prevent HIV infections in this era of apparently treatment-led epidemic management. Has prevention become a secondary concern? How is medicalisation affecting prevention technologies? What new formations of community, citizenship and activism now inflect prevention?

Such complexity intersects with local circumstances, underlining the tremendous challenge of reflecting on the global pandemic. A public discourse of HIV treatment possibility, twinned with treatment's unavailability, dominates in most developing-world contexts. Here, alongside expectations of improved treatment outcomes in well-resourced, mainly urban communities, access to full and first-line, rather than third world-'appropriate' treatment, is the primary demand of advocates and activists. As in the developed world, power in relation to treatment technologies is at issue – but the political rather than the medical shape of that power is foregrounded. UNAIDS' '3 by 5' programme, promising to provide ART for three million people by 2005, reached its target at the end of 2007. Today, treatment reaches four million people (UNAIDS, 2009a), under half those currently thought to require ART. The G8 and the African Union have pledged to provide 'universal' ART access by 2010; one of the Millennium Development Goals is to halt HIV's spread by 2015. These goals will be difficult to meet. Health and social care practitioners in the developing world face large challenges when implementing HIV treatment in highly resource-constrained circumstances and in an overall framework of postcolonial global exploitation. There is strong competition for HIV resources from other health, social and economic constituencies. Client requirements for food, education, employment and gender equity and non-violence often go far beyond HIV service providers' remit. International aid organisations' financial and practical provision varies not just with recipient organisations' performance, but also with national political positions. International pharmaceutical corporations resist expanding provision;

developed-world donor fatigue sets in. In the face of a raft of other economic, social and political difficulties, AIDS fatigue characterises many high-prevalence nations themselves. Developing-world HIV prevention programmes are also problematically situated, sometimes presented by international agencies as a kind of developing-world 'alternative' to treatment, often addressed outside the requisite broader cultural and development frameworks that nations with high HIV prevalence themselves emphasise. Currently, such programmes are tending towards medicalised yet patient-centred, low-technological initiatives such as microbicides and circumcision.

The advent of effective HIV treatment has sharpened focus on disparities in treatment access and delivery between different parts of the globe. However, similar disparities exist within countries, where refugees cannot secure fully-fledged citizenship and the related rights to health care, where racialised, sexualised, gendered and economically disempowered social groups experience HIV service exclusion, and where HIV service provision may differ radically between geopolitical areas and across urban and rural communities. The various histories and epidemiologies of HIV epidemics, different levels of prevalence, varieties of political ownership and response, and widely divergent resource availability also strongly differentiate prevention and treatment technologies.

Across all these situations, ART has nevertheless defined 'new', post-treatment or treatment possibility generations, emerging in the mid-1990s in the developed world and post-2003 in most developing countries. These generations differ widely in the medical and other resources available to them, but have some potentially shared assumptions about living with HIV and the 'risks' of HIV transmission. HIV positive people taking ART in the developing world are also now having experiences similar to those in developed-world countries living long term with HIV medication. However, in the developing world, this group continues to live alongside large numbers of people who need but cannot access ART, as well as large numbers of people newly infected each year. Moreover, effective treatment, or its possibility, arrived at very particular times within each epidemic. For instance, ART became available only after many HIV positive people in developed countries and some African countries, such as Uganda and Tanzania, had died. Within other low-resourced countries such as South Africa, where the epidemic developed later, this second, 'post-treatment' or 'treatment-possibility' generation involves people doing well on ART, living *alongside* many who are dying. This book reflects on these and other developments in the 'post-treatment' or 'treatment-possibility' period.

We are adamant that this book is not a tale of two pandemics, of the technological and economic haves and have-nots, of the ART-rich versus the ART-deprived, of high versus low prevalence, of prevention failure versus prevention success. Instead, we suggest that there are multiple, intercalated epidemics even within single countries. The possibilities of more effective treatment since the mid-1990s; an international commitment to developing-world treatment delivery since 2003; new approaches to prevention that address empowerment, especially women's empowerment; engagements with the prevention capabilities of treatment; and an increasing commitment to interrelating treatment with prevention have contributed to a distinct moment within the pandemic. This moment has different characteristics across developed and developing worlds and low- and high-prevalence contexts, but rests in all these cases on treatment possibility, alongside an increasing recognition of the long term, shifting and widely diffused character and effects of the pandemic.

Aside from changes in the technological governance of HIV and questions over how to engage properly with its global and local impacts, there have also been theoretical developments in the study of technologies and health that are significant for the HIV field. The intensified technologisation of healthcare raises questions concerning the 'lay' public's engagement with science and technology, and with increasingly scientised and managerial forms of governance. One set of concerns lies with how such managerial technologism reformulates relationships between the producers and consumers of healthcare, and the implications of this reformulation for the politics of expertise, and personal and 'human' security. There is a rapidly unfolding debate concerning how to frame and investigate these developments in theoretical and methodological terms. For example, perspectives such as the analysis of socio-technological assemblages (Rose, 2007), biosociality (Rabinow, 1999), health citizenship (Robins, 2009), political economy (Webster, 2007) and psychosocial analyses (Davis, 2009), among others, have been applied to technologies and health governance. In addition, current critical perspectives on health governance engage policy shifts that have come to enshrine the 'prudent', risk-averse individual as the prerequisite of all human agency (Fox and Ward, 2006; Ward et al., 2006). Such perspectives also challenge formulations of the neoliberal subject of governance that delineate 'health' through assumptions about individual rights and responsibilities. With different emphases, these approaches to health and technologies therefore take up concerns about governmentality as opposed to narrow notions of 'governance'.

That is, they address the discourses, practices and resources by which modern states generate governance by producing and controlling their subjects as citizens (Foucault, 1991).

We argue that social research on the technologised and transnational HIV pandemic has much to contribute to debates concerning health and technologies, in terms of empirical and theoretical insight and because of the local and global complexity that characterises the pandemic. The book thus provides a way to interrogate intensified processes of technologisation and transnationalism through the lens of HIV, with strong implications for discourses and practices of health governance in their broader substantive and theoretical contexts.

HIV technologies and social inquiry

There are many ways of taking social inquiry to health technologies. In this part of the introduction we would like to note several perspectives that the reader will identify in the chapters to follow or that help frame the overall argument of the volume, in order to make connections with wider debates concerning health governance. In particular, we make mention of analyses of the political economy of health technologies, recently discussed by Andrew Webster in his book *Health, Technology and Society* (2007). We also refer to the ways in which health technologies, and not least those used to treat and prevent HIV, have implications for risk calculus and identity (Adkins, 2002; Lupton and Tulloch, 1998). Many of the chapters draw on Foucauldian notions of governance as governmentality, and in particular Nikolas Rose's conceptualisation of biopolitics (2007) and to a lesser extent, Paul Rabinow's related articulation of biosociality (1999). For that reason we also make note here of some of the key aspects of these formulations of health governance. We also draw on Chantal Mouffe's (2006) conceptualisation of contested and multipolar politics, because of the ways in which this approach draws attention to the complexities of different biopolitical locations, so characteristic of the ART possibility era and its expressions in different parts of the world.

A key strategy for this volume that the reader will recognise throughout is its address to health technologies, and therefore HIV technologies, as socio-technical systems or assemblages, rather than as apparatuses merely surrounded and modified by social formations. This perspective on technologies as simultaneously the cause and effect of society is that outlined by Webster in his 2007 book. Health technologies can emerge inside the health field through the action of practitioners and patients, but they can also be produced less directly by medical researchers and pharmaceutical corporations' efforts to limit and control disease. Some technologies have origins entirely outside the health field but come to affect it, for example, information technologies from business and industry. Webster also draws attention to the 'who' of technological innovation. For him, the actors are multiple and all need to be taken into account to understand health technologies. Such actors include government, commerce, consumers, researchers and media. Analysis of these circumstances involves examining how the various actors of health technologies interact, what social effects they produce and the claims on knowledge and expertise that support such effects. Analysis can also take up struggles and conflicts over health technologies to spur their theoretical elaborations. As will become plain, many of the chapters in this volume draw on this approach to elaborate the social and governmental dimensions of HIV technologies.

Contemporary health technologies, including HIV technologies, are also seen by some analysts as linked with the focus on risk and risk management in health care (Lupton, 1999). Many of the biomedical technologies typically associated with HIV impinge on risk perception and more particularly risk behaviour. For example, one's sexual or drug-using practices might put one at risk of HIV infection. HIV treatment is itself suffused with risk calculations. For example, the ongoing management of ART relies on clinical markers such as CD4 counts, viral load and viral genotyping that are used to judge the risk of treatment failure and inform modifications of treatment. Questions of superinfection with drug-resistant forms of HIV are also couched in terms of risk for the person with HIV. Researchers and HIV educators have examined the extent to which the knowledge generated by ART and the blood tests used to support it influence risk behaviour (Elford, 2006). A central concept here is 'disinhibition', or 'treatment optimism' as it is sometimes called, which is the idea that the health benefits of ART reduce motivation to avoid risky sexual behaviours (Van De Ven et al., 2004). As has been argued however, such uses of risk are methods of governance. For Lisa Adkins (2002), risk is not so much a challenge for late modern subjects as a method by which such subjects come into being. According to Kane Race (2001, and also in this volume), the risk knowledge systems that proliferate in and around HIV treatment have the effect of drawing attention to the practices of people who use these technologies, particularly in connection with sexual relations and ART dosing. As many chapters in this volume demonstrate, a critique of dimensions of risk management is central to the analysis of HIV technologies.

The risk-related forms of subjectivity and requirements on sexual and drug-dosing practices noted by writers such as Adkins and Race indicate that biomedical HIV technologies are more than just substances and tools. While impinging on the action of the virus in bodies, they are also vehicles for social effects in the lives of people affected by HIV. By extension, it is also possible to argue that social practices are 'technological' in the sense of the effects they mobilise in and through materiality, bodies and social relations. This expanded notion of HIV technologies is important to this volume because it allows us to consider not only the various biomedical but also the social and governmental technologies that are used to address HIV. This perspective opens up the prospect that HIV technologies can be ostensibly biomedical as in ART, but also social, as in HIV prevention or care interventions. It also demonstrates that the various dimensions of technology are present in all attempts to address HIV, that is, ART is always a social and political treatment and HIV prevention has material mediations, expressions and effects. After all, HIV treatment and prevention are joined in the sense that they both address a viral entity and seek to operate on it. Furthermore, HIV is itself dependent on social relations and cultural practices, engagement with which is constitutive of all manner of HIV interventions including prevention, social care, assistance with treatment and dosing and ART adherence. Social inquiry about HIV must therefore address how the different aspects of its constitutive technologies coexist and articulate. Such inquiry allows us to question assumptions regarding the boundaries between technologies and permits an interrogation of HIV technologies themselves across the diversity, contradictions and fractures of their field. Many of the chapters in this volume draw on this expanded notion of HIV technologies as the basis for their arguments in relation to different aspects of HIV such as prevention, treatment and their intersection; or discourses of 'communication' and 'participation' that operate in both prevention and treatment programmes.

A concept that usefully illustrates the importance for HIV social research of constructing technologies in newly expanded ways is Rabinow's formulation of biosociality. This concept draws attention to the social relations that give rise to contemporary health technologies, but it is also able to describe the desired and sometimes unexpected or even counterproductive social effects of technologies. The concept emerged in Rabinow's ethnography of a French genetics research company undergoing rapid transformation in the 1990s (1999). Rabinow pointed out that health technologies such as genetic tests and therapies reveal surprising dynamics of alliance and conflict between interested parties, including those affected by genetic illness and their families, clinicians, researchers, venture capitalists, the popular media and government at local, national and, in his particular case, international levels. Rabinow also noted that as biomedical technologies are brought into being, their social ramifications are not all immediately intelligible. This perspective parallels one of the arguments of this volume pertaining to HIV technologies. As we will see, several chapters imply the changing nature of HIV technologies and the sometimes hidden effects of such changes.

One important insight derived from Rabinow's work is that the interrogation of health technologies necessarily extends to the assumptions that influence how they are used. For example, intersecting with the interests of this volume, Rabinow examined French responses to the threat of HIV in the blood transfusion economy as part of his ethnography of the genetics research company. He showed how in the French situation, abstract principles of the governance of the nation state made it hard to act to protect the blood supply from HIV. In particular, the French system relied on universalist notions of the inviolable rights of the blood donor to anonymity and the related valorisation of the gift and the gift-giver over and above the recipient and their rights. This 'sacralisation' of a particular social form immobilised attempts to prevent HIV coming into and circulating within blood transfusion products. Government officials were reluctant to act lest they be accused of transgressing what were seen as fundamental human rights to privacy and liberty, axiomatic to French nationhood and citizenship. According to Rabinow, such sacralisation is an example of how the (sometimes hidden) tensions that reside in forms of citizenship can feature in health technologies. As he noted in relation to the example of blood donation,

> The spiritual technology becomes its own worst enemy, activating a dangerous machinery that forestalls or inhibits the flourishing of things, practices, and assemblages that could well enhance and abet our search for a better form of life before they are either understood or communally evaluated through experience.
>
> (1999: 79)

Rabinow's comments with regard to HIV and blood donation suggest the salience of notions of biosociality for HIV technologies. This approach affords a way of investigating how HIV technologies are heavily inflected with citizenship concerns, for example, the negative effects of outmoded social forms, the clashing of multiple understandings of good government, the crisis for universalism in situations of rapid socio-technical change and the pursuant ethical challenges for individuals and collective practices.

This notion of the biosocial has wide implications and can also be usefully extended and differentiated to draw attention to its ramifications for social inquiry. Rose (2001: 22) has argued that through the science of new genetics and related technical and conceptual developments, we have entered the age of 'vital politics' and 'biological ethics' where increased capacity to exact biological control of human life brings with it intense political, social and ethical questions. This biopolitics can be seen in gene selection technologies that promise the control of disease among future populations or notions of permanent 'cognitive and affective enhancement' of the human species, as it is sometimes called (Savulescu, 2009). Biosociality is therefore not only a way of framing health technologies; but due to the far-reaching implications of socio-technological change, it can be used to provide a conceptual framing of contemporary society in general. In a recent paper, Rabinow and Rose (2006) suggest that this biological politics is at least fourfold. It involves 'truth discourses' most obviously, but certainly not exclusively in the biological sciences, and particularly, today, those which address humans' 'vital' characteristics as living organisms, and try to understand, predict, control and change them. Second, biological politics involves experts, who claim and are given legitimacy in investigating and proclaiming truth discourses, and the relations such experts have with the rest of us, who rely on their systems of knowledge. Third, biopolitics focuses on trying to improve people's health and by implication their whole lives, individually and within groups. The fourth aspect of biological politics concerns the means by which people try to make such improvements for themselves, by their own self-constitution as health-pursuing 'biosocial' or 'somatically individualist' subjects.

Contemporary health technologies, in the broad sense in which we have defined them, are the technologies of this biological politics. They are a specific subset of technologies in general: 'hybrid assemblages' (Rose, 2007: 17) of knowledges, practices, habits and material resources that have particular effects – in this case, in the field of health. Such health technologies are political: they are tied to collective and effective decision-making. They are ethical, that is, they pursue ideals of good conduct, though these ideals are often conflicting (MacIntyre, 1984; Rabinow, 2007). And they are importantly implicated with scientific knowledge, not simply suspended relativistically in a net of interconnected discourses and practices, but positioned in a close relationship to knowledges and strategies that improve and prolong lives (Hacking, 2006). HIV technologies of treatment and prevention demonstrate these complex relations clearly. They operate at different levels, from the international down to the local; they have different interests at each level, varying across fields of operation which range from medical research and practice through tactics of self-care to artistic production. They often contradict each other and they are nevertheless directed at having positive effects on people's lives as 'vital' subjects. Such complexities are reflected in the chapters in this volume.

Another aspect of biological politics that plays a significant role in this book is its transnationally differentiated character, something that can usefully be understood through Chantal Mouffe's (2006) formulation of contemporary politics' complex, struggled-over nature. The divergent status of low-, middle- and high-income countries in relation to health technologies is clear, particularly in the HIV treatment case. However such differences do not constitute the entirety of political engagement around HIV technologies. As Rabinow and Rose (2006) point out, 'biopower' cannot be equated with politics without becoming an overextended, empty and purely descriptive concept. Moreover, transnational differences in HIV technologies cannot be reduced to a simple opposition between 'global south' and 'global north' without neglecting the complexities of HIV technologies in these locations. People infected or affected by HIV are a transnational, sometimes globalised, but also highly differentiated group. Their differences appear on many intersecting axes – of for instance class, gender, sexuality, ethnicity, 'race', religion, and nation-state history and politics, as well as the histories and politics of each national epidemic, and individuals' own varying health statuses. It is not helpful to reduce such axes to the coordinates of imperialist postcolonialism.

Mouffe's understanding of multiple polarities and ongoing contest as constitutive of contemporary political formations allows us to understand HIV technologies in an appropriately complex transnational frame. From this perspective, such technologies cannot be associated with a single social group, a particular social level or a specific ethical orientation. They are, rather, heterogeneous, multi-levelled, and deployed in the service of many different moral discourses. Such a perspective allows us to analyse the contingency and particularity of HIV technologies.

The chapters in this book assume, for example, that variations between HIV policies within the developing and developed worlds are significant elements of biopolitical technologies, rather than trivial variations amongst the 'have-nots' and the 'haves' of biocapital. And they acknowledge that low-resourced people living with HIV in high-income countries, while they are disadvantaged within these HIV 'treatment-era' contexts, have importantly different relations to HIV technologies from HIV positive people in low-income countries. Despite structural disadvantage, they are distinctly developed-world subjects and citizens.

We also assert that analyses of HIV technologies need to extend to their psychosocial ramifications. Biopolitical inquiry does not often address the psychic interiority of citizens, or the memories, thoughts and emotions implicated in socio-technical transformations. When it is considered, subjectivity is commonly rendered as one reflection of biopower, or self-subjection to forms of pastoral power. In a much-quoted formulation, Rose (1996) describes subjectivities as Deleuzian 'infoldings' of technologies into interiority, a formulation that gives the psychosocial little particularity. In contrast, Mouffe's account (2006) provides for a psychosocial space constituted by symbolic and subjective disjunctions that are partially bridged by social and psychic efforts towards citizenship. Mouffe's analysis pays attention to psychosocial aspects of political processes: to the imaginings, metaphoric articulations and fantasies that support hegemonisation and democratisation alike. Butler (2005) similarly captures the subjectifying social and ethical interpellation of the self, alongside the powerful inextricability of lives from subjecthoods, while also suggesting that socio-political differences affect the subject's structuration at the most fundamental, symbolic levels.

Such insistence on the place of the psychosocial within political analysis is important for addressing HIV technologies. HIV research, especially research on the significance of medical technologies for people affected by the epidemic, is overwhelmingly preoccupied with the knowledge, thoughts, beliefs, behaviours and emotions of HIV citizens. Such research thus perpetually tries to identify, describe and modify unruly 'psychosocial' factors that disrupt or evade conventional HIV prevention and treatment technologies. Reflexivity about this 'psychosocial' field appears, in different guises, in all the chapters in this volume. The chapters' varying formulations work to map out the complexities and contradictions of HIV's 'psychosocial' technologies.

Overview of chapters

The chapters in this volume follow a sequence loosely arranged as so: case studies that address the governance of HIV prevention and treatment and the intersections of these, reflections on the subjective aspects of HIV technologies derived from close-focus qualitative research and investigations of HIV technologies that trouble scientific and ontological assumptions about HIV and how the epidemic should be governed.

Governing HIV treatment and prevention

In Chapter 2, Catherine Campbell examines four international aid organisation interventions in South Africa and Zimbabwe predicated on the concept of community participation. Drawing on social psychology and Foucauldian notions of networks of power and resistance, Campbell summarises what is known about how to conduct interventions effectively, delineating the approaches and methods that underpin what she refers to as 'AIDS competent communities'. Campbell shows that despite such knowledge, international aid agencies often sponsor disappointing interventions. Campbell shows that interventions designed to facilitate community participation, can actually exert their own power over communities, raising deep questions over the participatory aspects of these interventions. Programme failure is often rationalised in terms of external factors and rarely in terms of the conduct of the intervention itself. Ironically then, such programmes, ostensibly predicated on community participation and empowerment, find ways of explaining why they have not done what they set out to do in terms of the failings of communities themselves. Campbell argues that this paradox of development governance stymies effective HIV education and support interventions.

In Chapter 3, Fareed Abdullah and Corinne Squire present a case study of the rollout of ART in the Western Cape of South Africa. The rollout is regarded as an exemplary programme for HIV care in transitional country contexts. Abdullah and Squire identify and examine what conditions of the rollout made it successful. Drawing on Rose's notions of biopolitics, they show that effectiveness can be attributed to the community-wide dissemination of ART provision to primary care providers and engagement with community activists and lay counsellors. This chapter develops the concept of HIV citizenship as a way of addressing HIV technologies in the ART possibility era.

In the fourth chapter Eric Mykhalovskiy examines the history of a Canadian community-based organisation over the course of the HIV epidemic and particularly in relation to the advent of ART availability in the mid- to late 1990s. Mykhalovskiy uses this case to question the integration discourse used by government and other agencies to address the relationship between treatment and prevention in the ART era. The advent of ART has sponsored much controversy and debate concerning the impact it will have on HIV prevention. For some, ART is seen to displace prevention and therefore increases HIV transmission. Mykhalovskiy reverses this standard critique to examine how HIV prevention imperatives have impacted on, and in some cases arguably distorted, the purposes of HIV treatment. Mykhalovskiy shows how integration discourse is necessary given the effects of ART for the health of people with HIV. However integration discourse can also be counterproductive for people with HIV because of the way it works to strengthen responsibility for HIV prevention, among other effects. HIV prevention imperatives rob HIV treatment of its original justification as a way of restoring the health of people with HIV and replace it with a notion that ART is the means by which people with HIV can be governed to prevent transmission of HIV to others. Like Campbell, Abdullah and Squire, Mykhalovskiy creates an argument that, to moderate such effects, the practical experience and skills of community agencies need to be incorporated into this new HIV technology of integration.

HIV subjectivities

In Chapter 5, Lindy Wilbrahim writes about her work in South Africa exploring the discursive production of good parenting in relation to the HIV epidemic. Wilbrahim formed groups with parents to discuss a text extract from Lovelines, a regular column in popular magazines in circulation in South Africa. Lovelines addresses parents, encouraging them to reflect on their practices in an effort to encourage the prevention of HIV transmission in young people in South Africa. Using Foucauldian notions of discourse analysis, Wilbrahim discusses the classing and racing of parenting expertise, elaborating an account of good parenting as an HIV technology and reflecting on its benefits and drawbacks.

In Chapter 6, Paul Flowers draws on qualitative interviews with men and women with HIV residing in Scotland and England to address the psychosocial dimensions of living with HIV in the ART possibility era. Flowers provides a detailed picture of the physical, mental and relational challenges of HIV diagnosis and health maintenance. A key theme in his analysis is to question the discourse of normalisation emanating from epidemiological accounts of the ART era and how these marginalise the psychosocial experiences of people with HIV. This chapter therefore reflects the argument made by Mykhalovskiy in relation to the undesirable aspects of the mixing of public health imperatives with the effects of ART for people with HIV.

Also drawing on interviews, in Chapter 7 Mark Davis examines personal responses to the impact of ART on the risk of transmission in sexual practice. This chapter underlines the arguments of Mykhalovskiy and Flowers that epidemiological rationalisation of ART positions people with HIV uneasily at the intersection of treatment and prevention. Drawing on Rose's notion of 'informational biocitizenship', Davis explores the extra-technical aspects of ART-related knowledge and the implications for the ethics of sexual relating. This chapter shows how people with HIV address these challenges by drawing on their experiences of HIV-related self-care. Like Campbell and Wilbrahim, Davis argues for increased dialogue with regard to the uncertainties, confusions and challenges for sexual ethics that arise in and around the use of ART.

New epistemologies and ontologies

In Chapter 8, Race examines the controversy surrounding so-called barebacking among gay men and the related concept of serosorting. Barebacking coincides with the ART possibility era and has connections with the use of HIV antibody serostatus to determine 'like with like' sexual connections where condoms are not used for sexual intercourse because HIV transmission is not thought possible or significant. It also resonates with the general impact of ART on the status of HIV infection as a serious health concern, presumably making sexual intercourse without condoms seem less dangerous than it was and therefore enabling cultures of barebacking. Using a Foucauldian framing, Race reverses the typical discourse regarding barebacking to reveal how the striving for ethical, sexual relationality underpins the practice. Race therefore addresses barebacking as an HIV technology in its own right. He explores its dual status as both a form of autonomy on the part of some gay men with HIV and as transgressive of what is taken to be good HIV citizenship under the imperatives of HIV prevention. Race shows that this duality underpins behavioural research seeking to explain barebacking behaviour. He argues that useful research needs to be reflexive with this duality.

In the last substantive chapter in this volume, Marsha Rosengarten and Mike Michael examine the ethical controversies surrounding the clinical trials for pre-exposure prophylaxis (PrEP) in countries in Africa and Asia. PrEP is an experimental form of biomedical HIV prevention where those at risk of HIV transmission take ART on a regular basis to reduce the likelihood of HIV infection. PrEP is therefore emblematic of the overlapping of treatment and prevention technologies. Rosengarten and Michael examine clinical trials for PrEP as sites of enormous complexity for HIV governance with controversial and potentially unknowable effects combined with opportunities for using biomedical technologies in innovative and productive ways. Because PrEP is squarely a biomedical form of HIV prevention it is both harbinger of the new formulations of HIV technology and crystallises many of the themes raised in previous chapters. Rosengarten and Michael show how clinical trials of PrEP raise questions of citizenship, controversial engagements with local trial communities and the impact of ART on HIV prevention and vice versa. This chapter addresses the extra-material in HIV technologies and extends to a discussion of ethics and science and the ontological status of the HIV virus itself.

In the final chapter, Davis and Squire reflect on the arguments developed in each of the chapters and return to some of the key points raised in this introduction. We will focus on some cross-cutting dimensions that will appear in the chapters, in particular the clashing and synergies apparent in the articulations of HIV treatment and prevention technologies and struggles over truth claims that have significance in the governance of a treatment possibility epidemic. We will also reflect on the forms of HIV citizenship implied in transnational and local diversity and draw attention to the underlying 'pragmatics' that inform the chapters in this volume and that have relevance for future inquiry and intervention.

References

Adkins, L. (2002) *Revisions: Gender and Sexuality in late Modernity* (Buckingham: Open University Press).

Butler, J. (2005) *Giving an Account of Oneself* (Fordham, NY: Fordham University Press).

Centers for Disease Control (2009) 'HIV/AIDS surveillance report, 2007', online: http://www.cdc.gov/hiv/topics/surveillance/resources/reports/2007report/pdf/2007SurveillanceReport.pdf, accessed: 16 April 2009.

Davis, M. (2009) *Sex, Technology and Public Health* (Basingstoke: Palgrave Macmillan).

Elford, J. (2006) 'Changing patterns of sexual behaviour in the era of highly active antiretroviral therapy', *Current Opinion in Infectious Diseases*, 19, 26–32.

Foucault, M. (1991) 'Governmentality', *in* Burchill, G., Gordon, C. and Miller, P. (eds), *The Foucault Effect: Studies in Governmentality* (Chicago: University of Chicago Press).

Fox, N. and Ward, K. (2006) 'Health identities: from expert patient to resisting consumer', *Health: An Interdisciplinary Journal for the Social Study of Health, Illness and Medicine*, 10, 4, 461–79.

Global HIV Prevention Working Group (2008) 'Behaviour change and HIV prevention: [Re]considerations for the 21st century', online: http://www.globalhivprevention.org/pdfs/PWG_behavior%20report_FINAL.pdf, accessed: 16 April 2009.
Hacking, I. (2006) 'Genetics and the future of identity', *Daedalus*, Fall, 81–95.
Lupton, D. (1999) *Risk* (London: Routledge).
Lupton, D. and Tulloch, J. (1998) 'The adolescent "unfinished body", reflexivity and HIV/AIDS risk', *Body and Society*, 4, 2, 19–34.
MacIntyre, A. (1984) *After Virtue* (Bloomington: Indiana University Press).
Mouffe, C. (2006) *On the Political* (London: Routledge).
Peltzer, K., Niang, C., Muula, A., Bowa, K., Okeke, L., Boiro, H. and Chimbwete, C. (2007) 'Editorial review: Male circumcision, gender and HIV prevention in sub-saharan Africa: a (social science) research agenda', *Journal of Social Aspects of HIV/AIDS*, 4, 3, 658–66.
Rabinow, P. (1999) *French DNA: Trouble in Purgatory* (Chicago: University of Chicago Press).
—— (2007) *Marking Time* (Princeton: Princeton University Press).
Rabinow, P. and Rose, N. (2006) 'Biopower today', *BioSocieties*, 1, 195–217.
Race, K. (2001) 'The undetectable crisis: changing technologies of risk', *Sexualities*, 4, 2, 167–89.
Robins, S. (2009) *From Revolution to Rights in South Africa* (Durban: UKZN Press).
Rose, N. (1996) 'Authority and the genealogy of subjectivity', *in* Heelas, P., Lash, S. and Morris, P. (eds), *Detraditionalization: Critical Reflections on Authority and Identity* (Oxford: Blackwell).
—— (2001) 'The politics of life itself', *Theory, Culture and Society*, 18, 6, 1–30.
—— (2007) *The Politics of Life Itself: Biomedicine, Power and Subjectivity in the Twenty-First Century* (Princeton: Princeton University Press).
Savulescu, J. (2009) 'Should we use technology to change our genetic destiny?' *Monash University Faculty of Arts Public lecture Series, 16 April, Federation Square, Melbourne.*
UNAIDS (2009a) 'Letter to partners from UNAIDS Executive Director Michel Sidibé. February 26', online: http://www.unaids.org.cn/en/index/topic.asp?id=582&classname=News&class=2, accessed: 16 April 2009.
—— (2009b) 'Psychosocial support with PLWHIV. February 2', online: http://info.worldbank.org/etools/docs/library/250608/02%20Planning%20for%20support-Cherabi_English.pdf, accessed: 16 April 2009.
—— (2009c) 'AIDS Epidemic Update,' online: http://data.unaids.org/pub/Report/2009/2009_epidemic_update_en.pdf, accessed: 28 November, 2009.
Van De Ven, P., Murphy, D., Hull, P., Prestage, G., Batrouney, C. and Kippax, S. (2004) 'Risk management and harm reduction among gay men in Sydney', *Critical Public Health*, 14, 4, 361–76.
Ward, K., Davis, M. and Flowers, P. (2006) 'Patient expertise and Innovative Health Technologies', *in* Webster, A. (ed.), *Innovative Health Technologies, Health Technology and Society Series* (Basingstoke: Palgrave Macmillan).
Webster, A. (2007) *Health, Technology & Society: A Sociological Critique* (Basingstoke: Palgrave Macmillan).

2

Technologies of 'Participation' and 'Capacity Building' in HIV/AIDS Management in Africa: Four Case Studies

Catherine Campbell

Introduction

Sub-Saharan Africa carries the heaviest burden of HIV/AIDS. Marginalised groups are particularly heavily affected. Women and young people carry the highest burden of infection. Poor people and people in rural areas have the least access to health and welfare assistance. Millions of people are dying of what is in principle a preventable and treatable disease – often in conditions of almost unbelievable suffering – with no medical help at all. Against this background, people are increasingly referring to lack of 'political will' as the reason for the continuing grip of HIV in Africa. This is fast becoming a buzzword in debates. In the Executive Summary of the 2006 UNAIDS report, which pulls together the state-of-the-art deliberations of a range of international agencies, the final sentence reads: 'We know what needs to be done to stop AIDS – what we need now is the WILL to get it done' (UNAIDS, 2006: 24).

Discussions of political will in the media and academic literature often centre on 'corrupt' or 'incompetent' African leaders (Lewis, 2005), leaders of wealthy countries that contribute too little to international aid efforts (Attaran and Sachs, 2001; UNAIDS, 2008) or to economic actors in profit-hungry pharmaceutical companies (Bond, 1999; Heywood, 2002). This focus is part and parcel of a tendency to identify the operations of 'the political' in terms of the words and actions of high profile leaders. However, Foucault (1995) emphasises that power operates in a complex and multiple range of sites and channels, and should be investigated in the least obvious as well as most obvious of places. Following his advice, this paper is part of the author's wider project of highlighting the multiple sources and operations of power that shape responses to HIV/AIDS in sub-Saharan Africa.

Elsewhere we have examined the way in which power operates at a micro-level in remote rural communities in South Africa, looking at how relationships of gender (Campbell et al., 2006; 2007a) and generation (Campbell et al., 2007b; 2009) undermine the likelihood that poor rural people will make optimal use of both formal prevention, treatment and care services as well as informal sources of social support. We have also looked at the way in which the functioning of traditional leadership structures serve to undermine such access (Campbell and Gibbs, 2008a), and at factors that limit the responsiveness of district-level health and welfare agencies and personnel to the needs of the local communities they claim to serve (Nair and Campbell, 2008). At the symbolic level, we have examined the way in which representations of the HIV/AIDS struggle in the South African media serve to mask and undermine the massive role being played by poor women and households in shouldering the burden of HIV/AIDS (Campbell and Gibbs, 2008b).

The aim of this chapter is to examine the role of highly respected international development agencies, supported by armies of well-funded academics, in continuing to support and fund ineffective HIV/AIDS management programmes in Africa. How do these actors and agencies serve to contribute to the perpetuation of power inequalities in the guise of benevolent assistance? We address this question through discussion of four case studies of southern African care and prevention programmes in which we examine the contradiction between the rhetoric of 'community participation' and local 'capacity-building' – with all its implicit promises of empowerment and positive social change for marginalised people – and the reality of programmes which claim to implement these strategies.

Billions of dollars of international development aid have been poured into HIV/AIDS management in Africa. There have been some encouraging reversals in the epidemic's hold in some countries, for instance, Uganda and Zimbabwe (UNAIDS, 2008). However, there is little evidence that HIV/AIDS interventions have played a role in this. In fact in a recent randomised control trial of state-of-the-art interventions in rural Zimbabwe, it was found that HIV/AIDS incidence was actually *higher* in the intervention sites that had been targeted by prevention programmes than in the control sites that had not been targeted (Gregson et al., 2007). A key reason for the disappointing outcomes of many programmes is their failure to resonate with the perceived needs and interests of target communities (Campbell, 2003). As the UNAIDS report cited above acknowledges, 'Community involvement is essential if any of our grand plans are to be achieved' (UNAIDS, 2006). Yet agencies all over Africa are failing to facilitate proper community involvement in AIDS programmes – communities are systematically excluded from meaningful participation (Gruber and Caffrey, 2005; Rau, 2006).

Despite a great deal of international and regional policy rhetoric (African Union, 2006; South African Government, 2007; UNGASS, 2001) about the importance of community participation in AIDS efforts, the bulk of HIV/AIDS interventions are biomedical and behavioural in nature, targeting individual knowledge, skills or disease states, and imposed on passive communities by outside experts (Parker and Aggleton, 2003; Parker et al., 2000; Waldo and Coates, 2000). Within the specialist HIV/AIDS prevention literature, programme evaluations focus overwhelmingly on technical aspects of programme design and delivery, and characteristics of the target audience (Kippax and Van de Ven, 1998). The little attention that is given to the social relations that frame these interventions tends to focus mostly on the indigenous social relations in which programme beneficiaries are located, paying less attention to features of the health programme itself that might have undermined its effectiveness. Within the HIV/AIDS literature virtually no attention is given to the role which implementing organisations play in facilitating or hindering the effectiveness of HIV/AIDS programmes.

Development anthropologist David Mosse (2004) argues that programme failure is invariably constructed in a way that blames everyone except for the development agencies that implement programmes and the so-called 'expertise' that informs them. He comments that analyses of development failures overwhelmingly lay the blame on events, situations and people outside of the framework of development expertise and authority. In so doing, the inputs and actions of academics and development agencies are distanced from any responsibility. Ironically, rather than leading to critical reflection and change in the views and practices of experts and agencies, failures are explained in ways that reinforce the very agency–community relationships, and the very systems of expertise within which health projects are entangled.

The social psychology of participation

Our particular interest in the importance of community participation in HIV/AIDS programmes is driven by our starting assumptions about the social-psychological benefits of such participation (Campbell and Jovchelovitch, 2000). Here we explicitly position social psychology in opposition to health psychology. Health psychology tends to take the individual as its unit of analysis. Social psychology, by contrast, tends to take the individual–society interface as its unit of analysis. Mainstream health psychologists have been accused of playing an active role in driving the HIV epidemic through their persistent claims that HIV/AIDS can be prevented through behaviour change programmes targeting individuals (Waldo and Coates, 2000). While this might be the case in relatively affluent and educated populations in high-income countries (Johnson et al., 2002), this promise ignores the inescapable social dimension of the epidemic in many sub-Saharan African contexts.

Writing about AIDS in Africa, French anthropologist Didier Fassin refers to AIDS as the 'embodiment of history ... the way in which individual and collective histories are transcribed into individual and collective bodies' (Fassin, 2002: 65). In Africa, power relations of poverty, age and gender make it very difficult for many to protect sexual health. Ideally the epidemic would best be addressed through macro-social change leading to the redistribution of economic and political power, both locally and globally, but these are long-term goals, unlikely to be achieved in the near future. In the medium term, such efforts should be supplemented by the facilitation of programmes and processes that serve to buffer or ameliorate the impacts of social inequalities on peoples' health, through facilitating 'participation' by affected communities – viewing communities as one of the many sites through which social inequalities are imposed on individuals who respond in varying degrees of submission or resistance (Campbell, 2003; Howarth, 2001).

What kind of community participation is most likely to empower marginalised groupings to make the best use of prevention, care and treatment services, to change their own behaviour, and to provide support to others with HIV/AIDS? Participatory health programmes should provide people with the skills and knowledge they need to respond effectively to HIV/AIDS. These include not only directly AIDS-related skills in areas such as participatory peer education or home nursing, but also the development of local capacity in programme leadership and decision-making, so that people can play an equal role in shaping, implementing and evaluating programmes. People are most likely to feel they can take control of their health-related behaviour if they have experiences of being in control of other aspects of their lives (Wallerstein, 1992). Participation in programmes that are seen to elicit and reflect community views and needs, and to include community members in leadership and decision-making, is a key strategy for achieving this. The development of such skills and capacity among local people enhances the likelihood that grass roots communities will feel a greater sense of collective ownership of the problem of HIV/AIDS, as well as a sense of confidence that community members have both the individual and collective skills necessary to contribute to its management.

Ideally programmes should provide people with safe social spaces in which they can translate alien medical information into discourses that make sense to them and action plans that can be realistically implemented in the context of their lives. Such social spaces provide the possibility for critical thinking and dialogue (Freire, 1970; 1973). People are most likely to develop health-enhancing attitudes and behaviours when they have opportunities to engage in collective dialogue about the obstacles to behaviour change, and to brainstorm ways in which they might – individually and collectively – resist such obstacles. Interventions that take account of target groupings' understandings of the nature of a problem, and that strive to involve local people at all stages of devising and implementing strategies are most likely to resonate with the perceived needs and interests of the target groupings whose attitudes and behaviours they seek to change.

Such spaces also provide people with a sense of solidarity, common purpose and collective responsibility for contributing to the fight against HIV/AIDS. These hopefully serve to counter a sense of fatalism in the face of the enormity of the problem, and a passive sense that the problem is the exclusive responsibility of outsiders (for example, from government or NGOs) – and that local individuals and groups have no role to play.

Finally, programmes should provide the opportunities for community members to identify and build relationships with outside support agencies – in the NGO and public sectors for example – that have the political and economic influence to assist them in achieving health-related goals. Marginalised communities often lack the power to tackle serious health problems without substantial outside support ('bridging social capital').

Elsewhere we have argued that effective participation should result in the development of six psychosocial characteristics of what we call an 'AIDS competent community context'. This is a social environment in which grassroots people are able to work collaboratively in supporting one another to achieve behaviour change, stigma reduction, support for people with AIDS and their carers, support for volunteers and health workers responding to AIDS, and the accessing of health services and welfare grants where these exist. The six characteristics include appropriate knowledge and skills (including both AIDS-related and leadership skills), social spaces for dialogue and critical thinking, a sense of solidarity and common purpose, a sense of ownership of the problem and responsibility for tackling it, a recognition of individual and collective local strengths for leading and implementing a local response, and strong bridging relationships with outside support agencies (Campbell et al., 2007b).

From a social-psychological perspective there is no doubt that concepts and strategies of participation and local capacity building have a crucial role to play in the development of AIDS-competent communities and in enabling the success of health and social development efforts in marginalised contexts. However the paper will illustrate how these concepts may be hijacked by health and development experts, who pay lip service to them in programme and grant proposals, but fail to implement them effectively in practice. In this respect, the hijacked concepts of participation and capacity building could arguably be said to serve as disciplinary technologies (Foucault, 1977), implemented by the international development apparatus and part and parcel of the 'procedural applications of power ... through institutionally operated systems of intelligibility and control' (Hook, 2007: 216). According to Hook (2007: 216), a technology may be understood as 'an expert system comprised of a discrete set of applied skills, practices, knowledges and/or forms of specialist language, used, whether by experts on deviant subjects, or by individuals on themselves, as means of achieving objectives of increased mastery or control'.

Case studies

Against this background, this chapter looks at four international development programmes the author has been involved in evaluating in various contexts in southern Africa. Each project explicitly claimed to be community-led and community-owned, and was driven by an 'empowerment via participation' methodology. The aim of this discussion is to focus on some of the subtle ways in which each project served to exclude the types of community participation and empowerment most likely to facilitate health enabling individual and social change. It is framed within the context of Foucault's (1982: 152) injunction to focus on the more subtle manifestations of power, what he calls 'the meticulous rituals of power', operating in hidden and subtle places not always immediately evident to the more casual observer.

Ekuthuleni Youth Peer Education Project

The first of these is a youth peer education programme in the peri-urban community of Ekuthuleni, located near Durban, where one in ten 15–24 year-olds were HIV positive. Funded by a major Australian international funding agency, and administered by a powerful international Christian non-governmental organisation, it sought to limit HIV transmission through delivering youth-led peer education programmes. The author conducted a detailed case study of the programme, involving interviews and focus groups with a range of community representatives and programme employees (Campbell et al., 2005). The aim of the case study was to identify factors serving to facilitate or hinder the programme's success in increasing youth awareness of the dangers of HIV/AIDS and promoting health-enhancing sexual behaviour change. This was the only formal HIV/AIDS-related programme in the community, and local people were tremendously appreciative of the existence of the programme in principle. As the funders themselves acknowledged, however, the programme was having little impact on youth sexual behaviour in practice.

Our evaluation highlighted a number of ways in which the programme fell short of its claims to be community-led and community-owned. The programme proposal was developed by overseas 'experts', with little consultation of local people and a minimal sense of local 'ownership' of the project. The programme was run by black South African project workers – whose task was to train local youth to be peer educators. However, while project workers came from a similar ethnic background to local Ekuthuleni residents, they were not themselves local people. They lived outside of the community and drove in and out every day to do their work. The local community perception of project workers as 'outsiders' and their resentment that local people had not been considered for paid project posts, undermined the development of any sense of local solidarity with programme goals. There was little transfer of educational or organisational skills from the project's paid workers to local people. Finally, for a variety of complex reasons, the project had little success in building partnerships with public sector health and welfare organisations, or with related NGOs in the region.

As a result, when the project's international funders withdrew after the three-year period specified on the programme proposal, the programme collapsed, in the absence of any local ownership, skills or support networks to sustain it.

Entabeni 'barefoot doctors' AIDS-care project

The second programme was located in a remote deep rural area of Entabeni in northern KwaZulu-Natal in South Africa. Here 35 per cent of pregnant women are HIV positive (Barron et al., 2007). This project – funded by a major North American AIDS funder – had two goals. Its first goal was to train 'barefoot' volunteer community health workers to provide AIDS care in remote rural community which had limited access to formal health and welfare services. This strategy of 'shifting' of tasks from health professionals to trained lay community members in underserved low-income settings is now a pillar of international AIDS policy (WHO, 2008). Its second goal was to build local and regional support networks for the volunteer team, consolidated into a 'partnership' committee that would sustain the volunteers' work over the long term once the project's three-year funded period ended. Furthermore, the project sought to use HIV/AIDS as a springboard to the wider social development of the community.

Contrary to the previous project, members of the Entabeni community were fully involved in the two-year development of the project proposal. Furthermore, the funders were exemplarily non-directive regarding the project's activities. In principle, they were content for the project to evolve in its own organic way, adapting to local needs and conditions, and allowing for time and funding to enable it to build up long-term relationships and support networks. The project has had some significant successes in training a cadre of competent volunteers who have delivered home-nursing and counselling support to large numbers of AIDS-affected households (Campbell et al., 2007a).

However, project facilitators are increasingly conscious of the more or less subtle ways in which the funders have imposed their own technical template on the way in which the project conducts and evaluates its work. The timing of the project has been completely at the mercy of the overseas funders' bureaucratic procedures and delays, with no sense of accountability to the beneficiary community. The donor agency has insisted on a 'numbers reached' form of project evaluation, which excludes any recognition of the importance of the community building agenda of the work.

Furthermore, project staff have battled with what they regarded as unrealistic demands for reporting and evaluation, which took no account of their resource and training limitations. Three overworked project staff spent a significant proportion of their time writing up to seven different funding reports a year, and responding to a range of difficult technical questions (for instance about levels of 'knowledge retention' in the community), which they were not qualified to answer, and which bore little resemblance to the project's community-strengthening goals which had been carefully negotiated with local people over a two-year period, and which the funders had accepted in their initial awarding of the grant.

Summertown mining industry project

The third example is drawn from an HIV prevention project in the gold mining community of Summertown, near Johannesburg (Campbell, 2003). This project was generously funded by a range of major British and North American development and research agencies. Here again, despite its claims to involve grassroots community groups (in particular migrant mineworkers, commercial sex workers and young people) in project management, there were various ways in which community members were excluded from significant participation.

Firstly, the conceptualisation of the project was dominated by needs and interests of researchers and funders – who defined project interests and activities in biomedical and behavioural terms, despite ample evidence (from the outset) that social factors would undermine biomedically and behaviourally driven efforts. Secondly, project management was 'top heavy' with medically oriented researchers and scientists, who had no expertise in programme management, health systems development or community liaison, all of which were essential to core project functioning. Finally, as the project gained status in the international donor community, members of highly respected Northern aid and research agencies engaged in distasteful professional turf wars over ownership of research options and findings, with agency staff invariably prioritising their organisations' interests over those of the poor communities they claimed to be assisting.

Within project discourse, the concept of 'community' was manipulated in such a way that target communities were effectively excluded from meaningful involvement in project decision-making. When members of the project's management committee used the term 'community' to denote the managers or agents of the changes the project sought to facilitate, they tended to refer to the relatively elite and powerful stakeholder representatives, such as biomedical researchers or representatives of the senior mine management. When they used the term 'community' to refer to targets of change, they tended to refer to the mineworkers, sex workers and township residents. Within project discourse, 'participation' referred to nothing more or less than community volunteers delivering unpaid HIV prevention services. Over time, local township residents became dissatisfied with what they perceived as the project's top-down managerial style. Ironically it was the community's festering anger at being treated as 'objects' rather than 'subjects' of the project's research component that eventually derailed the community-strengthening component of the project, leaving project management in the hands of traditional biomedical and behavioural researchers and practitioners who were not familiar with the community development ideals that had informed the project in the first place.

Kumahuswa home nursing project

My final example involves a home-based care club, set up and managed by an internationally funded NGO, in a small rural community in Zimbabwe. Here again, a so-called community empowerment programme was 'imposed' on the community by an outside agency, there was no local involvement in any aspect of project design, implementation or management, and what was referred to as community 'capacity building' focused on training poor people to provide unpaid welfare services to the community, rather than involving them in programme decision-making or leadership.

This was particularly clearly illustrated in an interview with the Chair of the club. She was an energetic woman, and she and five peers worked enthusiastically to provide the only formal support available to people with AIDS in the community. They distributed food parcels and blankets to AIDS-affected households, helped them provide nursing care for people dying of AIDS and met fortnightly to timetable their work and provide one another with support and encouragement. However, despite their dedication and commitment, it was clear that they knew nothing about the context of this work, or the organisation that facilitated it.

> 'They no longer bring the blankets and the food parcels, I am not sure why.'
>
> 'I am not sure who initiated this group.'
>
> 'We (the five women) don't network with anyone besides each other.'
>
> 'We have run out of gloves and we need a refresher course.'
>
> 'I am not sure of the future plans of this group because I am not part of the management.'
>
> Anna K., cited in Nhamo and Campbell (2009)

Conclusion

In debates about political will, organisations implementing programmes in sub-Saharan Africa usually assume that it is others that must change – others such as 'problematic' African leaders or 'promiscuous' community members. It is the argument of this chapter that as members of external organisations (in our roles as academics and development practitioners, for example) we are equally complicit in development failure in more subtle ways. There is an urgent need for us to look at how our *own* actions and practices contribute to disappointing programme results.

The case studies outlined above seek to highlight ways in which the practices of development agencies may often run directly counter to processes of empowerment and capacity building that are necessary preconditions for more effective HIV prevention and AIDS care. Too often, discourses of 'participation' and 'community mobilisation' are used as a smokescreen for programmes in which local people are used to provide unpaid welfare services according to an externally imposed agenda, but quite systematically excluded from any meaningful involvement of the type that would facilitate health-improving social-psychological changes.

Here it needs to be emphasised that facilitating genuine and effective community participation is not easy. Furthermore proper community 'buy-in' and grass roots engagement in health programmes is only one of several necessary preconditions for success. Elsewhere, for example, we have argued that marginalised communities are unable to solve major health problems without strong support from outside agencies (Nair and Campbell, 2008). However, in the absence of meaningful involvement of communities, little can be done to help the most HIV/AIDS vulnerable groupings. Studies repeatedly cite proper community participation as vital for effective prevention, accessing of services, treatment and care.

Discussions of the complexities of implementing effective community engagement, and of the failure of generations of development programmes to bring about sustainable reductions in poverty and ill health, tend to generate both pessimistic and optimistic conclusions. These depend on the ways in which different commentators conceptualise power. Those who view power as a monolithic entity, possessed and wielded by the strong against the weak and powerless, tend to conclude pessimistically. Such commentators suggest that the failure of so-called 'development' programmes – funded by rich western countries and implemented in poor countries – is part and parcel of the on-going and systematic perpetuation of global inequalities.

Prominent among this group is Escobar (1995: 39) who argues that the history of the relationships between rich and poor countries is structured in such a way that 'it has created a space in which only certain things can be said or even imagined'. In short it enables only the saying and imagining of forms of 'community participation' that systematically exclude the possibility of effective community involvement, and of the development of leadership capacity among the world's poor and dispossessed. These involve nothing more or less than 'the collapse of social emancipation into social regulation' (Escobar, 2004: 213; Cooke and Kothari, 2001). In a similar vein Kitching (1989: 195) comments that 'Development is an awful process. It varies only ... in its awfulness.'

More optimistic commentators shy away from what they argue is a simplistic and one-dimensional account of power as a force held by some groups and not others, and used by the former to retain their unambiguous hold on power over the latter. They reject what they identify as the implicit dualism between all-powerful international development agencies and powerless impoverished Africans. Citing Foucault, they argue that power can be productive as well as repressive, and that wherever power is wielded, there lies the possibility of resistance. Within this vein, Lewis and Mosse (2006: 10) argue that 'reality is messy ... [and that] encounters between developers and people tend to be much more complex and nuanced than meets the eye'.

What might this mean in the context of the case studies outlined above? Frederick Douglass (cited in Seedat, 2001) argues that 'power is never conceded without a demand', and that elite groups seldom hand over power without vociferous demands from the excluded. Perhaps it is the case that even flawed projects of the kinds discussed above give members of marginalised groups a glimpse of the possibility of playing more active and empowered roles in their social and public lives. This might include women, young people, rural people and the poor – the groups most disproportionately affected by HIV/AIDS in Africa. Such glimpses might even be important though veiled milestones on the long road of building the skills, confidence, networks and platforms for making the 'demands' that Bulhan speaks of in increasingly assertive and effective ways over time.

This chapter has focused on the technologies of participation and capacity building in the context of HIV/AIDS management in four economically deprived southern African settings. Much remains to be learned about the way in which various elements of this paper's analysis would be relevant to HIV/AIDS work with socially excluded groups in other low- and high-income contexts. Furthermore, the focus of this particular chapter has been HIV prevention and AIDS care, with none of the four case study communities having access to antiretroviral drug treatment at the time of writing.[1] However preliminary studies suggest that wherever possible, prevention, treatment and care need to go hand in hand for optimal outcomes (Achmat and Simcock, 2007). Furthermore it is very likely that meaningful community participation will be an important influence on treatment success in marginalised settings, given that treatment access and adherence is heavily affected by community-level factors such as AIDS stigma, and the social and cultural appropriateness of services (Campbell et al., 2005; Coetzee et al., 2004).

Acknowledgements

Thanks to Derek Hook and Andy Gibbs for discussion of various points.

References

Achmat, Z. and Simcock, J. (2007) 'Combining prevention, treatment and care: lessons from South Africa', *AIDS*, 21, Suppl. 4, S11–S20.

African Union. (2006) *Addis Ababa declaration on community health in the African region* (Addis Ababa, Ethiopia: African Union).

Attaran, A. and Sachs, J. (2001) 'Defining and refining international donor support for combating the AIDS pandemic', *Lancet*, 357, 9249, 57–61.

Barron, P., Day, C. and Monticelli, F. (2007) *The district health barometer – year 2006/7* (Durban, South Africa: Health Systems Trust).

Bond, P. (1999) 'Globalization, pharmaceutical pricing, and South African health policy: managing confrontation with U.S. firms and politicians', *International Journal of Health Services*, 29, 4, 765–92.

Campbell, C. (2003) *Letting them die: how HIV/AIDS prevention programmes often fail* (Bloomington: Indiana University Press/Oxford: James Currey/Cape Town: Doublestorey).

Campbell, C. and Gibbs, A. (2008a) 'Facilitating HIV/AIDS "empowerment" programmes within traditional authority structures: experiences from southern Africa', submitted.

—— (2008b) 'Representations of HIV/AIDS management in South African newspapers', *African Journal AIDS Research*, 7, 2, 195–208.

Campbell, C., Gibbs, A., Maimane, S., Nair, Y. and Sibiya, Z. (2009) 'Youth participation in the fight against AIDS in South Africa: from policy to practice', *Journal of Youth Studies*, 12, 1, 93–109.

Campbell, C. and Jovchelovitch, S. (2000) 'Health, community and development: towards a social psychology of participation', *Journal of Community and Applied Social Psychology*, 10, 255–70.

Campbell, C., Maimane, S. and Sibiya, Z. (2005) 'The impact of social environments on the effectiveness of youth HIV prevention', *AIDS-Care*, 17(4), 471–8, May 2005.

Campbell, C., Nair, Y., Maimane, S. and Sibiya, Z. (2005) 'Home based carers: a vital resource for effective ARV roll-out in rural communities?', *AIDS Bulletin*, 14, 1, 22–7.

—— (2007a) 'Building contexts that support effective community responses to HIV/AIDS, *American Journal of Community Psychology*, 39, 3–4, 347–63.

Campbell, C., Nair, Y. and Maimane, S. (2007b) '"Dying twice": towards an actionable multi-level model of the roots of AIDS stigma in a South African community', *Journal of Health Psychology*, May, 12, 3, 403–16.

—— (2006) 'AIDS stigma, sexual moralities and the policing of women and youth in South Africa,' *Feminist Review*, 83, 1, 132–8; special edition on sexual moralities.

Coetzee, D., Boulle, A., Hildebrand, K., Asselman, V., Van Cutsem, G. and Goemaere, E. (2004) 'Promoting adherence to antiretroviral therapy: the experience from a primary care setting in Khayelitsha, South Africa', *AIDS*, 18, Suppl. 3, S27–S31.

Cooke, B. and Kothari, U. (2001) *Participation: the new tyranny?* (London: Zed).Cornish, F. and Campbell, C. (2009 This should read 2009 'The social conditions for successful peer education: a comparison of two HIV prevention programmes run by sex workers in India and South Africa', *American Journal of Community Psychology*, 44, 123–35.

Escobar, A. (1995) *Encountering development: the making and unmaking of the third world* (Princeton: Princeton University Press).

—— (2004) 'Beyond the Third World: imperial globality, global coloniality and anti-globalisation social movements', *Third World Quarterly*, 25, 207–24.

Fassin, D. (2002) 'Embodied history: uniqueness and exemplarity of South African AIDS', *African Journal AIDS Research*, 1, 1, 63–8.

Foucault, M. (1977) *Discipline and punish: the birth of the prison* (Harmondsworth: Penguin).

—— (1982) 'The subject and power', in H. Dreyfus and P. Rabinow (eds), *Michel Foucault: beyond structuralism and hermeneutics* (Brighton: Harvester Press).

—— (1995) *Power/knowledge: selected interviews and other writings, 1972–77* (London: Longman).

Freire, P. (1970) *The pedagogy of the oppressed* (Harmondsworth: Penguin).

—— (1973) *Education for critical consciousness* (New York: Continuum).

Gregson, S., Adamson, A., Papaya, S., Chimbadzwa, T., Mundondo.J., Nyamukapa, C., Mason, P., Garnett, G., Chandiwana, S., Foster, G. and Anderson, R. (2007) 'Impact and process evaluation of integrated community and clinic-based HIV-1 control: a cluster-randomised trial in eastern Zimbabwe', *PLoS Medicine*, 4, 3, 0545–55.

Gruber, J. and Caffrey, M. (2005) 'HIV/AIDS and community conflict in Nigeria: implications and challenges', *Social Science and Medicine*, 60, 6, 1209–18.

Heywood, M. (2002) 'Drug access, patents and global health: "Chaffed and waxed sufficient"', *Third World Quarterly*, 23, 2, 217–31.

Hook, D. (2007) *Foucault, psychology and the analytics of power* (Basingstoke: Palgrave Macmillan).

Howarth, C. (2001) 'Towards a social psychology of community', *Journal for the Theory of Social Behaviour*, 31, 2, 223–38.

Johnson, W., Hedges, L., Ramirez, G., Semaan, S., Norman, L., Sogolow, E., Sweat, M. and Diaz, R. (2002) 'HIV prevention research for men who have sex with men: a systematic review and meta-analysis', *AIDS*, 30, Suppl. 1, S118–29.

Kippax, S. and Van de Ven, P. (1998) 'An epidemic of orthodoxy? Design and methodology in the evaluation of effectiveness of HIV health promotion', *Critical Public Health*, 8, 4, 371–86.

Kitching, G. (1989) *Development and Underdevelopment in Historical Perspective*, 2nd ed., Routledge: London.

Lewis, D. and Mosse, D. (2006) 'Encountering order and disjuncture: contemporary anthropological perspectives on the organisation of development', *Oxford Development Studies*, 34, 1, 1–13.

Lewis, M. (2005) *Addressing the challenge of HIV/AIDS: macroeconomic, fiscal and institutional issues*, Center for Global Development Working Paper No. 58. http://www.cgdev.org/content/publications/detail/2730/, 30 April 2009.

Mosse, D. (2004) *Cultivating development: an ethnography of aid policy and practice* (London/Ann Arbor, MI: Pluto Press).

Nair, Y. and Campbell, C. (2008) 'Building partnerships to support community-led HIV/AIDS management: a case study from rural South Africa', *African Journal AIDS Research*, 7, 1, 45–53.

Nhamo, M. and Campbell, C. (2009) 'Social capital and the "HIV competent community": a case study of community responses to HIV/AIDS in rural Zimbabwe', submitted.

Parker, R. and Aggleton, P. (2003) 'HIV and AIDS-related stigma and discrimination: a conceptual framework and implications for action', *Social Science and Medicine*, 57, 1, 13–24.

Parker, R., Barbosa, R. and Aggleton, P. (eds) (2000) *Framing the sexual subject: the politics of gender, sexuality, and power* (Berkeley: University of California Press).

Rau, B. (2006) 'The politics of civil society in confronting HIV/AIDS', *International Affairs*, 82, 2, 285–95.

Seedat, M. (ed.). (2001) *Community psychology: theory, method and practice* (Cape Town: Oxford University Press).

South African Government. (2007) *HIV and AIDS and STI strategic plan for South Africa, 2007–2011* (Pretoria: South African Government).

UNAIDS. (2006) *2006 Report on the global AIDS epidemic: executive summary* (Geneva: UNAIDS).

—— (2008) *2008 report on the global AIDS epidemic* (Geneva: UNAIDS).

UNGASS. (2001) *Global crisis – global action* (New York: UN).

Waldo, C. and Coates, T. (2000) 'Multiple levels of analysis and intervention in HIV prevention science: exemplars and directions for new research', *AIDS*, Suppl. 2, S18–26.

Wallerstein, N. (1992) 'Powerlessness, empowerment and health: implications for health promotion programmes', *American Journal of Health Promotion*, 6, 3, 197–205.

WHO. (2008) *Task shifting: global recommendations and guidelines* (Geneva: WHO).

Notes

1. Currently only one-third of those who need antiretroviral drugs in sub-Saharan Africa have access to them (WHO, 2008).

3

Technologies of Treatment: Scaling up ART in the Western Cape, South Africa

Fareed Abdullah and Corinne Squire

Introduction

This chapter examines technologies of 'treatment scaleup', the extension of antiretroviral treatment (ART) to most or all HIV positive people who need it, in the Western Cape, South Africa. The chapter describes three technologies related to ART scaleup: those of administration; partnership, rather different to the 'partnership' Campbell (this volume) describes and thirdly what we refer to as treatment citizenship. These non-medical treatment technologies operate alongside conventional medical treatment technologies to make up a successful, even exemplary, ART scaleup. The chapter also argues that the success of these technologies derives from their involvement in a larger phenomenon: a new construction of 'HIV citizenship' within the Western Cape.

The Western Cape's ART programme, begun in April 2004, was the first treatment scaleup to high levels of provision within a high-prevalence low-resourced context. At the time, many politicians, policymakers and clinicians thought that delivering ART programmes in such settings was dangerous or impossible. Today, the programme's success and influence, particularly for other developing-world scaleup programmes, is widely acknowledged (World Health Organization, 2007). The Western Cape's earlier demonstration projects, starting in 2001 in the township of Khayelitsha, near Cape Town (Coetzee et al., 2004), were important models for the World Health Organization (WHO)'s '3 by 5' programme, aiming to provide ART to three million HIV positive people by 2005 – a goal met two years late (see http://www.who.int/mediacentre/factsheets/2003/fs274/en/ and World Health Organization, 2006). The first author of this chapter headed Western Cape AIDS programmes from 1996 to 2005, and directed the scaleup

(Abdullah, 2004, 2006; Abdullah et al., 2006; Boulle et al., 2008). He now works with the Global Fund to Fight AIDS, Tuberculosis and Malaria, as Africa Unit Director, again with scaleup a priority. The second author conducted interviews about HIV support with HIV positive people in the Western Cape between 2001 and 2004, when many interviewees were beginning or contemplating ART (Squire, 2007). This chapter draws predominantly on the first and to a lesser extent on the second area of work.

How did particular technologies deliver the Western Cape scaleup? This chapter takes technologies to be 'hybrid assemblages' (Rose, 2007: 17) of knowledges, practices and material resources that have particular effects. In this case, they are directed at enabling people with HIV-related illness to be healthy, happy and socially active. The 'hybrid' diversity of the administrative, partnership and treatment citizenship technologies examined here renders them heterogeneous; they intersect with and sometimes contradict each other. And power does not lie only with the technologies' makers and controllers. Their natures, applications and ownership are contested by everyone involved with them.

Administrative technologies are rarely examined in accounts of HIV treatment. Lacking clear or appealing politics, they usually appear simply as bureaucracy. However, they can have important political effects, as well as treatment effectiveness, depending on how their ownership is structured. In this chapter, they counter the instances Campbell describes of determining and surveillant, top-down bureaucratisation. Partnership technologies, often present solely in the discourse of the more powerful partners, can also be to some extent delivered in practice – as Campbell's chapter demonstrates, and this chapter reiterates. What we are calling 'treatment citizenship' technology is harder to describe, lying in the fields of education, social dialogue and community action. Elements of it are however frequently identified as contributing to the success of HIV programmes. In the Western Cape scaleup, treatment citizenship's effectiveness is very clear.

The chapter suggests that these technologies worked within a larger frame of developing discourses and practices of 'HIV citizenship'. This concept has some important precedents. Rabinow (1996) describes a 'biosocial' realm of collectively articulated experience and organisation, through which human subjects engage critically and sometimes effectively with discourses of post-nineteenth century biopower (Foucault, 1980). Rose (2007: 134) frames this 'collectivising moment' as one aspect of 'biological citizenship'. Such citizenship, constituted by individualising biopower, allows some space for subjects to wrest some power for themselves, individually and collectively, on the basis of their 'vital interests'. Rose cites HIV activism as an example of biological citizenship; others include genetic citizenship, bioinformational citizenship and biopolitical citizenship generally, a category into which HIV activism may fall. Robins (2008) frames South African HIV activism as 'health citizenship', a description that attends both to the country's radical constitutional guarantee of health care for all, and to the necessarily integrated nature of health care activism in developing-world contexts, where access to all medical care, not just ART, is restricted, and where health is undermined by hunger and poor infrastructure as well as disease. Robins focuses on HIV activists, for whom making connections between HIV and other issues is central to political effectiveness. Our concern with the Western Cape ART programme, however, takes in the whole of the province's HIV positive population, even those with little connections to non-medical services; addresses the specificities of HIV treatment needs and makes attention to *HIV* citizenship more appropriate.

Citizenship for an HIV-infected or affected person has to be constructed in relation to the particularities of HIV: its fatal or, since the mid-1990s, potentially chronic character; its stigmatisation and associations with socially 'transgressive' sexualities and drug use; its national significance in high-prevalence countries, particularly in sub-Saharan Africa and its global politics which imbricates all HIV positive people in transnational as well as local debates. These specific characteristics, as well as the more general health and biological components of HIV citizenship, shape HIV technologies like those driving the Western Cape's scaleup.

Despite the success of the Western Cape programme, problems remain. There are difficulties of sustainability, accountability and democracy in the programme's systems, as well as in its local, national and international governance. Treatment does not work for everyone, has side effects and may need to change periodically. It also produces fresh challenges in people's lives as HIV becomes a long-term but still-stigmatised and potentially fatal illness, with new implications for employment, family roles and sexual relationships. In epidemics where prevalence and incidence (annual new cases) remain high, as in South Africa, the economic future of ART is hard to guarantee without factoring in effective prevention; treatment's relation to prevention is also much debated. Universal ART can have resource-diverting implications for other public services, particularly health, and for the voluntary sector. The successful scaleup technologies and discourses and practices of HIV citizenship described in this chapter do not circumvent the problems of 'development' Campbell adumbrates when discussing 'partnership' and 'capacity building'. Western Cape scaleup experiences also indicate that novel 'psychosocial' issues continually arise. Nevertheless this chapter suggests that the Western Cape scaleup demonstrates the possibility of treatment technologies operating effectively in high-prevalence, low-resource contexts, as part of broader formations of HIV citizenship, pragmatically aligning effectiveness with medical and political hope.

The next sections of the chapter describe the context and nature of the scaleup, before examining the three technologies, and their current and future limitations.

ART: A 'universal' technology?

One of the UN Millennium Development Goals is to 'combat HIV/AIDS, malaria and other diseases' and halt HIV's spread by 2015 (http://www.un.org/millenniumgoals/). The UN, G8 and African Union pledge treatment and care for HIV to 80% of those who need it, and 25% reductions in HIV prevalence, by 2010. Four million people are now thought to be taking ART (World Health Organization, 2009), the most effective medical treatment for people with serious HIV illness – up from 400,000 in 2003 (World Health Organization, 2006). This medical treatment technology has powerful consequences, markedly decreasing HIV mortality and prolonging life. In the developed world, many HIV positive people are now living in their second decade of treatment. When treatment is generally available, people access it when they are healthier and are more likely to do well (Boulle et al., 2008). When HIV positive people on ART have unsafe sex, there is less likelihood of them transmitting HIV. When HIV positive women on ART have children, those children are less likely to have HIV (Jackson et al., 2007). Expanded treatment also reduces the pandemic's psychosocial, economic and political effects – especially significant for high-prevalence epidemics in sub-Saharan Africa. By turning HIV from a fatal condition into a manageable, if difficult, chronic illness, ART reduces stigma (Wolfe et al., 2008) and enables disclosure (Skogmar et al., 2006) and this in turn encourages testing, and others' early, successful treatment (Chesney and Smith, 1999). ART means less strain on health services, more people working, more parents looking after children, fewer orphans. It ameliorates the lives of some of the most disadvantaged people in the world. Its absence, and communities' resulting decimation by HIV, can lead to powerful social and political disaffection.

'Universal' ART provision is hard to attain. It is economically, institutionally and socially difficult to implement, and the pandemic, the virus and treatment itself are uncertain and changing. ART is prohibitively expensive, particularly those second-line and later variants not available as generics, for high-prevalence low- and middle-income countries. These countries are therefore positioned as perpetual aid recipients, sourcing a significant share of ART's cost from international donors such as PEPFAR (President's Emergency Plan for AIDS Relief) and the Global Fund. As epidemics 'mature' and more people get ill, as new infection rates remain high, as HIV diverts or is perceived to divert resources from additional important health and other basic needs and as international NGOs back-pedal on or struggle to meet – depending on your perspective – their universal treatment commitments, ART's sustainability is often questioned. ART is also said to be potentially enabling transmission by presenting HIV as a manageable chronic illness, untransmissible when treated (Davis, this volume), turning it into a medicalised, technologically determined condition, and obviating HIV prevention, without which the possibility of universal treatment recedes further.

An early objection to universalising treatment in developing-world epidemics was that complicated medications could not work for resource-deprived people, adherence would be poor and resistance would grow. However, adherence is higher in developing- than developed-world epidemics, and adherence-related resistance is low (Boulle et al., 2008). Another objection is that 'gold-standard' ART treatment programmes, medically on par with the developed world and providing 'wraparound' social services, are divisive resource misuse. However, such programmes are not viewed as over-provision in their own context. Similarly, the organisation Partners for Health, responsible for innovative HIV treatment in Haiti and Malawi, opposes dual-track care, suggesting treatment 'should be both medical and moral ... based on solidarity, rather than charity alone', involving 'everything that the providers would do for their families – or themselves' (http://www.pih.org/who/vision.html).

Do the difficulties of universal treatment mean that there will continue to be 'us' and 'them' HIV epidemics, distinguished by ART access and the lack thereof? This chapter argues that we are living neither with two treatment-differentiated epidemics, nor in the 'post-crisis' situation described in some developed-world communities with treatment access (Rofes, 1998) but rather in a stage characterised by universalised HIV knowledge, including treatment knowledge, but uneven provision and expectations. This is still a 'treatment possibility' rather than a 'treatment' era. This stage nevertheless raises some common debates across the diversity of national epidemics, about how ART technologies, as well as HIV care, education and support technologies, are working, and how they could operate better.

Scaling up ART in a high HIV-prevalence province

South African addresses to treatment technologies are instructive to consider since the country has high prevalence – 16% among adults (UNAIDS, 2008) – and more people on treatment than any other nation. Despite great economic diversity, South Africa is a middle-income nation, with relatively well-developed health services and infrastructure in urban and peri-urban areas. Today between 28% and 42% of the approximately 900,000 people estimated to need treatment, are receiving it (World Health Organization, 2009; Republic of South Africa, 2008). In 2004, when the Western Cape province's ART scaleup began, there were no government plans to provide ART. In a reconstructing country faced with five million people dying from HIV-related illnesses within a decade, and with relatively good internal and external resources, treatment seemed to many as both an ethical necessity and an economic and practical possibility.

In 2004, the Western Cape decided to make ART, previously restricted to a small number of sites, available to all the people in the province who needed it. Currently around two-thirds of those thought to need ART in the province, are taking it. On conservative calculations, 72% of the first adult and 85% of the first child patients, many of whom started treatment when very sick and who came from a highly mobile peri-urban population, are still in the programme (Boulle et al., 2008). Life expectancy when they started was at most one year.

At the beginning of scaleup, Western Cape HIV prevalence in the Western Cape was estimated at 200,000–300,000 out of a 4.2 million population (http://www.capegateway.gov.za/eng/your_gov/305). Ten to twenty per cent needed ART according to WHO guidelines on treatment. HIV affects fewer people, proportionally (13%, from antenatal screening) and in absolute numbers, than in other South African provinces, because of the population's higher socioeconomic status and because the most HIV-affected, black-African community in South Africa constitutes a relatively small fraction of the Western Cape population. However, antenatal prevalence in some districts reaches 33%. The province's resources, better overall than those of others, are low in rural areas, posing considerable scaleup challenges in some heavily affected districts. The health service suffers chronic understaffing, poor management and organisation, and lack of computerisation. There are eight million visits per year to clinics and four million visits per year to community health centres (Abdullah et al., 2006); by 2010, 25% will be for HIV (Abdullah, 2004).

Demonstration ART programmes at innovator sites had early success in the province in 2001 (Coetzee et al., 2004), building on the success of Prevention of Mother-To-Child Transmission, or PMTCT, programmes which the provincial health department had begun in 1998. After court action by activists against the government, who said it would be unworkable and too expensive, these successful, cheap and popular PMTCT programmes rolled out nationwide, albeit slowly, from 2001 (Moodley et al., 2003) but PMTCT was accessible throughout the Western Cape by 2003. Currently, Western Cape transmission rates for HIV positive women are 6.1% (Draper et al., 2007). The province's early-adopted and rolled-out PMTCT programmes formed an important treatment literacy foundation for patients and staff, particularly in the early stages of the ART scaleup.

By April 2004, when the national ART plan was implemented, the Western Cape already had 16 ART sites, treating 2327 people with Stage IV HIV illness or CD4 counts below 200 per mm^3 – a fourfold increase over the previous six months (Coetzee et al., 2004; Western Cape Department of Health, 2006). The province then rolled out ART to all major towns at 43 sites, two-thirds in primary care settings. Seven thousand to ten thousand people died in 2005 without accessing ART, but by March 2006, numbers had reached 16,234 adult and child patients on treatment – 65% coverage for both groups (Boulle et al., 2008). Figures for 2008 doubled, at 37,500 (Uys, 2008).

Criteria for success in the Western Cape ART programme are high levels of patients retained in care, and high levels of viral suppression among those patients. At the end of scaleup patients' first year on treatment, 75% had a CD4 count above 200 cells/mm^3. This figure increased to 86% at two years and 95% at four years on ART. Viral load tests showed 88% of adult patients achieving virological suppression after a year on ART and 85% showing suppression after four years. In this treatment-naïve population, virological suppression could be expected; but the rate is still very good in comparison with other rich and developing countries. Deaths in the first six months of treatment are now half what they were initially, as less-ill people seek treatment. Seventeen per cent of patients are on second line therapy after four years (Boulle et al., 2008).

ART's expansion and success in the Western Cape demonstrate ART scaleup's feasibility in resource-constrained settings. The scaleup started in a situation of low national HIV resourcing and education; relatively low levels of local health and social resources; low government commitment; patchy international commitment, pre-Global Fund and the numerically largest national epidemic with still-increasing incidence. In such circumstances, scaleup success merits attention. How did it happen?

In the Western Cape programme, pre-ART care for people living with HIV is provided mainly at local clinics and comes predominantly from nurses, who conduct voluntary counselling and testing, provide care for minor ailments, give ongoing counselling, and are responsible for regular checkups including six-monthly CD4 counts. Community health centres or district hospital outpatient departments initiate and maintain ART. HIV services, particularly ART programmes, always work with local NGOs and community-based organisations (CBOs). How this occurs, depends on agreements between specific health facilities and the organisations. These agreements involve HIV prevention and education NGOs and CBOs, as well as those focusing on ART literacy and support, and NGOs and CBOs with other remits such as counselling, advocacy, income generation, homecare and childcare. ART clinics, support services and PMTCT programmes are located close together, usually in the same building. ART delivery is always accompanied by education and counselling or peer support. It includes encouragement to disclose to at least one person in the patient's home environment. Again, its specific nature is determined by clinicians and NGOs or CBOS, but the programme emphasises 'psychosocial' factors such as understanding and accepting HIV status; 'positive' ways of living with HIV in sexual relationships, in having children and in nutrition, exercise and drug and alcohol consumption; and family and friendship network disclosure and support. There are strict protocols for patient recruitment, medication, and monitoring ART and other health progress, sometimes exceeding WHO guidelines. There is a firmly guaranteed supply of ART drugs, not easy where ART provision depends significantly on international donors. There is good additional care – secondary referrals for TB, immune reconstitution disease and major side effects – which enables good adherence. There are special arrangements for children, and for patients who are pregnant or who have psychiatric issues. Partnerships with national and international NGOs are actively pursued (Abdullah, 2004).

Political technologies of scaleup

We might expect, from South Africa's political contests around HIV and the country's politicised recent history, that ART scaleup would involve political technologies: explicit contests over power relations. However, as the above description indicates, there were no explicit political alignments within the programme. Political commitment from national leaders is often declared critical in tackling HIV epidemics, as in Uganda and Botswana (Epstein, 2006). In 2004, South Africa's governing ANC exhibited considerable disengagement from HIV. The Western Cape's political unpopularity at national level, because of its privilege and conservatism and the ANC's weaker position there, paradoxically enabled provincial support of ART scaleup and even of treatment HIV activism such as that of the Treatment Action Campaign (TAC). Later, as national health policy shifted towards ART scaleup, the Western Cape gained the position, highly unusual for this province, of national exemplar.

It might seem likely that the Western Cape scaleup's success drew on grass roots traditions of political activism derived from the anti-apartheid struggle. This link is, though, hard to substantiate. Some NGO, CBO and health service workers and volunteers involved in the scaleup had participated in the anti-apartheid struggle, left politics and in lesbian and gay activism; most had no such histories. Moreover, many of the health and social service professionals, civil servants, politicians, advocates and activists involved were too young for their efforts to be understood as a direct legacy of anti-apartheid struggle. The indirect legacy of this struggle for South Africa's HIV campaigns is indeed significant (Robins, 2008). It is possible, too, that the Truth and Reconciliation Commission's high-profile disclosures enabled HIV activism in the Western Cape's relatively politically open context. However, in the context of the Western Cape scaleup, these legacies were only part of a multi-level technological network.

Administrative technologies of scaleup

The technologies of the scaleup can be understood as first of all administrative rather than political governmentality. The scaleup's managerial sophistication has often been noted as distinguishing it from other provinces' programmes (Abdullah, 2004; Beresford, 2004). Administration acted as a kind of politics in itself, counteracting the simplifications and paralyses produced by 'politics-first' approaches to the pandemic demonstrated well by Campbell (this volume). Like conventional political technologies, this administrative technology involved decision-making and promoting change. Administration – a term derived from a word for 'service' – became, in the scaleup, a patient-centred, patient-serving political strategy.

The scaleup was planned by health department officials in consultation with clinicians and international, national and local NGOs. In addition to following WHO protocols and providing referrals for difficult issues, the health department asked clinics to develop broad psychosocial guidelines across all aspects of the programme. For instance, some selection guidelines addressed clinic attendance, successful TB treatment, treatment literacy and substance abuse issues. Support guidelines focused on adherence issues, but also less immediately relevant concerns such as relationships. The structure and content of psychosocial support does not seem to have affected ART outcomes, but support perceived as well-administered was judged to perform best (Infectious Disease Epidemiology Unit/ Department of Health, 2006).

The province put special effort into working with pharmacological services on drug sourcing and distribution. Previous province health initiatives had not addressed these services, but they were key for a programme depending on a rapid increase, province-wide, in drug availability; on imported drugs involving complex ordering and processing; on low-supply, high-demand drugs liable to 'leak' from the system and on a treatment protocol opposed by government and therefore liable to experience national-level administrative delays. The province also instituted programme-wide 'basics first' monitoring of patient retention, progress, amount and rate of antiretroviral drugs used, and – via treatment waiting time guidelines – care quality. This thorough and painstaking monitoring required already hard-worked professionals to keep additional detailed handwritten records. More complex data were collected from 'sentinel' sites with electronic access (Boulle et al., 2008; Western Cape Department of Health, 2006. The data were powerful ripostes to arguments about the impossibility of making ART treatment work in generalised high-prevalence low-resource epidemics. Some procedures and data turned out to be unnecessarily cautious and detailed. Adherence and loss to follow-up, addressed and defined more strictly than in developed-world programmes, proved less than expected, and viral rebound rates have not been high (Boulle et al., 2008). However, such 'overadministration' was a highly effective strategy, rendering the programme politically impregnable and building commitment to and confidence in it among patients and staff.

The politics of biocapital (Sunder, 2006), an economic form dedicated to extracting surplus financial and epistemic value from the 'vital' properties of living organisms (Rose, 2007), tends towards the minimum, quickest-achievable standards of administrative care, that will substantiate the value rather than the shortcomings of biological science. The administrative technology of this biocapital roll-out was by contrast highly cautious and regulatory. It shared, however, one common characteristic of biocapital development: rapidity.

Speed was important to reach people in this escalating epidemic, to try to reduce transmission through education and lower infectivity by treatment, to get treatment to people when they were at manageable numbers and before it was too late for them, and to establish treatment structures for the larger numbers who would need them later. To achieve this, the programme's management structures had to be rapidly effective. From the beginning, they had to provide drugs consistently, and to sustain an infrastructure that would let drugs be prescribed and taken effectively, encouraging adherence and minimising the development of resistance. Speed was promoted by putting policy and planning targets into the annual budget: the budget itself became a scaleup tool. Often this involved informed approximations (Abdullah, 2004). The programme had to estimate numbers of patients by site and then allocate appropriate budgets for drugs and labs, counsellors, nutrition, community and psychosocial support. Though in 2003 drug supply in ART-prescribing clinics was still patchy, the programme's parallel-systems approach to drug ordering, distribution and monitoring, had by the end of 2004 regulated supply. The programme also quickly mobilised Global Fund resources that became available from 2003; rapidly recruited and trained staff, for instance nurses and counsellors with ART-specific knowledge; and continually expanded their resource drive. Again, results were not immediate; in 2003–4 doctors dealing with ART in then-operational clinics were overwhelmed with patients, and staffing levels are still hard to maintain. The programme also quickly constructed appropriate infrastructure, including building and expanding clinics, starting with initiator sites which were receiving the most referrals. Finally, to work well, the scaleup had rapidly to establish consensus with all 'stakeholders' or partners: patients, local communities, CBO,s, HIV activists, interested national and international NGOs, and medical professionals at every level. From the beginning of the scaleup, resources were devoted to managing these partnerships so they could have rapid outcomes (Abdullah, 2006). One cannot scale up quickly, alone.

The detail, breadth and speed of the scaleup's administrative technology constituted a micro-politics of the epidemic. It set up participants in the scaleup – patients and staff – as citizens functioning within the HIV epidemic: as HIV citizens with specific means of ensuring access to and effectiveness of treatment. However, some of this technology's elements, for instance the strong collaborations which guaranteed its speed, were also components of other key technologies in the scaleup.

Partnership technologies

Technologies of partnership were central to scaleup. 'Partnership' is a problematic matter, rarely as easy to establish or as equal as it proclaims. It is often invoked in HIV and development discourse, where commitment to it can be a condition of receiving funding (Heywood, 2004), but ignored or exploited in practice. Campbell's chapter provides many southern African examples of partnership discourse without practice. In other South African provinces it has been questionably successful in supporting scaleup, particularly early on (Beresford, 2004). The Western Cape scaleup also generated examples of the difficulties of national government, local government and civil society partnerships. However, it demonstrated that it is possible to build associations of different and differently powerful 'stakeholders' in limited, contingent partnership working for specific goals around HIV treatment. In the Western Cape, such associations were essential for operational reasons, to deliver the medical and 'psychosocial' aspects of HIV treatment within resource-constrained circumstances, as well as ideologically, to promote a 'positive spiral ... where all parties were working together to do their best' in a programme seen to be 'innovative, responsive and inclusive' (Abdullah, 2004: 258). Such associations construct another important level of citizenship in the HIV epidemic, building that citizenship's relationships and identities as well as its effectiveness.

The Western Cape already had high levels of HIV 'partnership'-derived cultural and social 'capital' – HIV knowledge and social associations – that enabled ART scaleup partnerships. For instance, PMTCT knowledge and practices encouraged ART literacy and enrolment from the start of scaleup. With only 33% of pregnant HIV positive women enrolled in such programmes worldwide, largely because of low antenatal clinic attendance (UNAIDS, 2008), many countries cannot draw on such pre-existing sociocultural capital. Some other South African provinces also have much lower antenatal HIV testing rates (Republic of South Africa, 2008). Scaleup was further enabled by province expertise derived from earlier ART trial and demonstration projects, and related collaborations between clinicians, researchers, local health officials, and international and national NGOs and CBOs. Unlike programmes in many other high-prevalence epidemics, the Western Cape scaleup could cite such existing effective partnerships when making funding applications: a considerable strength.

However, scaleup could not rely on pre-existing partnerships to deal with the numbers requiring treatment across the whole province. The Department of Health had to create a generalised technology of partnership across all levels and sites of medical engagement. The scaleup devolves ART, often considered too complex and resource-intensive for primary health care environments, hence viewed as draining resources from and devaluing them, to precisely these environments, which are involved, too, in the programme's planning and monitoring. The scaleup's universal provision also lets primary-sector medical professionals address HIV much more effectively than before. Pre-scaleup, they were often reported as stigmatising, unhelpful and fatalistic (Squire, 2007). These reactions might be attributable partly to lack of treatment education (Beresford, 2004); partly to the 'deskilling', frustrating and depressing effects of being unable to access proven effective treatment for fatally ill patients. In 2002, a doctor was fired from his government job for allowing prophylactic ART prescription to raped women. By contrast, the medical alliances promoted by the Western Cape scaleup support highly motivating partnerships in cutting-edge HIV treatment and care.

Partnership also extends to new professional groups. Pharmacists are specifically addressed as active scaleup partners (Naimak, 2006). 'Lay' HIV counsellors, mostly with no prior medical or psychological expertise, are trained to support people on ART at a maximum ratio of 1:30, either visiting patients at home, giving onsite one-to-one counselling or facilitating onsite groups – much as counsellors work with support groups on PMTCT programmes. Treatment expansion functioned for existing lay HIV counsellors, as for medical professionals, as a powerful incentive, turning their previous role of dispensing comfort and nutritional advice into one of providing effective medical referrals, alongside information and socio-emotional support for 'living positively'. The partnership between lay counselling and the scaleup, building up a new, salaried profession of considerable size, has involved some economically motivated compromises. Status differences between lay counsellors and nurses remain controversial, with the former paid by private companies tendering to the province's Department of Health, and therefore lacking health department benefits: holiday and sickness pay, unemployment insurance. This differential promotes turnover, constrained however by unemployment rates of over 50% in the townships, informal settlements and rural areas where most counsellors live. As in this case, partnerships are never relations between exact equals. They involve negotiation towards contingent, pragmatic consensuses, often hard-won, on specific issues at particular times.

The scaleup encourages but does not mandate partnership between medical facilities and local NGOs and CBOs. It asks them to collaborate in deciding and delivering support mechanisms. Some sites initially even made joint clinican–NGO or CBO decisions about which patients to admit to the first stages of roll-out. The chosen method of education – collective or individual – and adherence support – onsite or in the community, one-to-one or in a group, counsellor-led or facilitated by family and friends – appears not to affect outcomes significantly. However, collaboratively agreed-on provision seems important, given less favourable outcomes in other settings that provide support less systematically, for instance, through GP practice (Abdullah, 2004; Infectious Disease Epidemiology Unit/Department of Health, 2006). In addition, the province's failure to exceed two-thirds provision may relate partly to NGOs' continuing struggles to deliver the education and support they aim for.

Involvement in scaleup gave NGOs and CBOs, too, new impetus. For example, some CBOs providing homecare were able to go beyond palliative care for the first time. In this high-prevalence epidemic, almost all CBOs' and NGOs' remit now includes HIV, precipitating multiple partnership possibilities. However, non-HIV-related NGOs and CBOs may be excluded from the new resources that scaleup brings, and external funders' requirement that applicants prioritise HIV can skew their work. For instance, Western funders frequently ask proposals on child poverty and abuse, and gender-based violence, to foreground HIV. The Western Cape provincial government has addressed this issue by expanding work in these areas in addition to its HIV programmes.

The scaleup's commitment to partnership also means that the programme aims to build the provincial health system generally, alongside HIV care. Many health professionals are themselves HIV positive, so health services gain directly from HIV treatment. More generally, full scaleup is impossible in poorly serviced areas and at primary health care level, without wholesale health system improvements. HIV's high demands on health services throughout sub-Saharan Africa have led to the mainstreaming of this double-track approach. Its implementation is not entirely successful. The Western Cape's failure to exceed two-thirds ART provision seems partly determined by continuing local health system deficits. Recent increases in patients lost to follow-up (Boulle et al., 2008) may indicate a system reaching capacity.

Partnership technologies can also offer an important alternative to the dichotomisation of HIV treatment and prevention. Treatment is often criticised as a diversion from prevention, supplanting it in policy, obviating considerations of prevention in HIV activism and in people's everyday lives (Davis, Mykhalovskiy; this volume), and abrogating scarce resources in the developing world. Though UNAIDS emphasises the necessary synergy of the two, HIV treatment is still often seen as creating divisions within health systems and stripping resources from prevention, which is associated less with scientifically validated, prestigious, drug-driven and resource-intensive technologies, and more with behavioural technologies. The Western Cape's 'partnership' technology however means that scaleup is delivered alongside treatment literacy; prevention resources such as condoms; support for safe sex negotiation, particularly for women; and general HIV education. This partnership is seeded by the educative effects of PMTCT programmes, particularly since these programmes reach almost all reproductive-age clinic-attending women. A related partnership, between scaleup and testing, has both prevention and treatment implications. As in other epidemics, testing became justifiable once treatment was available. On the back of universal PMTCT and the ART roll-out, antenatal testing rates have risen to 94.8% (Draper et al., 2007).

Declining HIV incidence and rising HIV awareness among younger people, and rising age of sexual debut especially among young women (Flisher et al., 2006) – with figures better than in other South African provinces – suggest the effectiveness of the Western Cape scaleup's technology of treatment and prevention 'partnership'. While the province's early comprehensive treatment programme marks it out, that programme seems to work alongside its integrated address to prevention, to constitute an important, social level of active HIV citizenship in people's sexual talk and actions.

Campbell vividly describes the difficulties of building partnerships, even within well-resourced and committed HIV prevention and education programme. Often, 'partnership' operates largely at the level of discourse. The Western Cape programme does not however rely on discourse or voluntaristic practice, but devotes considerable resources to fostering and managing partnerships at every level. In some situations, Campbell describes how HIV is not a personal priority 'owned' by all stakeholders, and how partners are separated by prohibitive geographical and social distances. In the Western Cape scaleup, the recognition of strong common interests between partners was promoted from the start through a concurrent public education programme, and peer education in schools, constructing the province's high levels of HIV cultural capital. Partnership is also fostered by the programme's decentred processes, carried out by primary health care facilities, nurses, counsellors and NGOs clustered together within highly affected neighbourhoods: everyone is close to the programme. Finally, perhaps most importantly, the promotion of treatment *with* education and prevention by the provincial health department, radically encourages partnership. HIV technologies that do not or cannot address the condition first as one that needs medical treatment, undermine their rationale by ignoring their own medical definition of their object, however much they are able to address other aspects of the condition.

The partnership-dependent delivery of ART, related prevention resources, and education for both treatment and prevention works horizontally and vertically, to develop social and cultural 'capital' (Campbell, 2003) within and across differently powerful groups: medical professionals; local politicians and officials; NGOs; CBOs; and community members who are patients, clients, service users and activists. These partnership-derived biosocialities of the epidemic are also part of a more broadly and actively articulated HIV citizenship, operating within and between these groups. For instance, drawing on ART programme partnerships, the Western Cape has supported campaigns against gender-based violence, a phenomenon linked to the epidemic in many ways (Jewkes, 2009). In these campaigns, HIV citizenship works both vertically, in partnerships between HIV-related CBOs, the health department and international donors; and horizontally, in partnerships between HIV positive women and men, and between people of different HIV statuses with common concerns about gendered violence and abuse.

Partnership technologies can only go so far. HIV programme ownership is not, as Campbell notes, spontaneously shared; there is always a struggle. Building bridging social capital between individuals and organisations with differential access to resources depends on addressing this discrepancy. The Western Cape scaleup has achieved an effective partnership technology that built HIV citizenship, not just through the partnership technology itself, but also through its commitment to a specific technology of HIV treatment citizenship, that addressed power relations directly. Treatment citizenship is a constitutive element of all HIV citizenship in the era of treatment possibility. In the Western Cape scaleup, however, the formations of representation and action that make up HIV treatment citizenship have a particular role.

HIV treatment citizenship

The Western Cape scaleup deploys a technology of HIV treatment citizenship that is less explicitly planned than the other technologies and harder to measure or record, but that is frequently remarked on in commentaries on the programme (Robins, 2008). This treatment citizenship technology is characterised by people's self-representation and action as members of HIV collectivities. The collectivities present as political, in the sense that they contest the power relations of HIV treatment, through education, social dialogue and activism.

Some treatment citizenship technology is easily apparent as such. For instance, the Khayelitsha ART demonstration project assessed applicants partly on the basis of their involvement with local HIV CBOs, at this point largely oriented towards treatment activism. Active treatment citizenship was thus a treatment criterion. The scaleup's implementation partnerships with NGOs and CBOs quickly also became partnerships with campaigners and activists. More generally, some patients, relatives and friends engaged strongly with medical and political institutions from the start, as in other epidemics (Epstein, 1996), demanding first treatment for opportunistic infections, then PTMCT, then ART, then specific medications not available within local or national protocols or supply chains. Many such campaigns appeared most strongly and first in this province, though the treatment-activist engagement of people throughout South Africa, especially via TAC, has been strong (Naimak, 2006). Robins (2008) describes this activism as a form of health citizenship, pursuing the rights guaranteed within the famously progressive South African constitution, which upholds the principles of Batho Pele – People First – and a 'better life for all'. He points to the strategic use of rights discourse within TAC which managed to articulate demands for ART in a national context of 'AIDS denialism', and in a language shared with the international governance discourse of the WHO and UN (see also Mbali, 2005).

However, across the Western Cape scaleup only some patients and fewer doctors participated in campaigning assertions of treatment citizenship. Activism is just the most visible face of treatment citizenship technology; the specificities of the condition necessitate other forms as well. HIV's stigmatisation and perceived transgressiveness consistently constrain activism. HIV's treatment normalisation may also divert activism, as in developed-world countries (Davis, Flowers, Mykhalovskiy; this volume). However, the difficulties of living with high-prevalence HIV, low resources and variable ART access, as in South Africa, differently limit activist commitment. The other kinds of treatment citizenship technology that play a part in the Western Cape's scaleup are HIV education and HIV sociality.

Treatment education, driven by the possibility of treatment even before treatment was available, has been integral to the scaleup's treatment citizenship technology. The province expanded ART education in parallel with scaleup, and some treatment literacy is required of all patients starting ART. Even in 2001, well before national education programmes on the issue, let alone ART or indeed other treatment availability, there was some province-wide education on treatment, as well as testing, healthy living and prevention – by NGOs, CBOs, popular media and the province itself. The province's roll-out of PMTCT programmes also educated people who, seeing the healthy babies of HIV positive women, started to demand the drugs for themselves. ART literacy in the Western Cape at the beginning of scaleup seemed relatively high. Even in 2001, HIV-infected people in the main peri-urban area had relatively good levels of knowledge of ART and other drugs (Squire, 2007).

Much treatment education was informally pursued, not formally delivered. Given government criticism of ART as exploitative and toxic, knowledge of it had to be wrested from competing sources of information. Patients' unexpectedly high levels of adherence often seems related to this self-educated engagement. Anecdotally, many clinicians report that people taking ART know the names of their drugs, alternatives available, and possible side effects, to a much greater extent than patients living with other chronic conditions such as diabetes and heart disease. Actively pursed, contested education thus seems a powerful aspect of the Western Cape's treatment citizenship, as it has been elsewhere. As is sometimes argued of Uganda (Epstein, 2006), HIV began stabilising when many within the epidemic became active, educated 'HIV citizens'. In the Western Cape, this happened first in the treatment, rather than prevention, arena.

Educated treatment engagement has spread outward from the Western Cape, particularly to family members living elsewhere. For instance, in the group of those 'lost to (treatment) followup' in the scaleup, a term which might suggest uncommitted or disorganised patients, many show high treatment commitment, and treatment planning. Some pregnant HIV positive women, for example, made their way to the Western Cape from other provinces with great difficulty, since they had no cash income for transport, to access its PMTCT programme. Other women and men, similarly cash-poor, came to the province to stay with family members and pursue their own treatment. Later, as treatment expanded for instance in the Eastern Cape, and as PMTCT babies were doing well, some patients returned home and thus were 'lost'. Currently, the scale-up's success means many patients feel free to move between medical facilities – moves which make care-retention statistics in a paper-based system, difficult to keep.

If treatment education was informal and contested, how did it work so well? The key route reported by Squire's (2007) informants, suggested by Campbell et al. (2007) in their accounts of developing 'HIV competence' in South African rural settings, and also indicated by accounts of the effectiveness of support and counselling groups (Hutchinson and Mahlalela, 2006; Flowers et al., 2006) involves not just obtaining knowledge, but also safe and open HIV sociality. This route recalls Rabinow's (1996) formulation of 'biosocial' collectivities organised around contested biological subjectivities. There is a possible, though not inevitable, association between such sociality – which also helps constitute, for instance, the 'partnership' technology, described above – and the broader identifications and actions of treatment citizenship. Campbell et al. (2007) also specify that HIV competence involves owning the virus socially as 'our problem', through the horizontal social–capital linkages described earlier as part of politicised partnership; and social effectivity. This account comes close to a Freirian programme for generating social change through collective critical dialogue (Freire, 1973). Western Cape treatment protocols, from the demonstration projects on to the scaleup, clearly embedded citizenly ART understanding and effectivity within sociality. They asked for NGOs, CBOs, and family and friends' involvement. Many required the participation of a familial or friend 'treatment assistant'. Building on the Western Cape demonstration projects, WHO ART scaleup guidelines also emphasise community and family support.

In ART scaleup discourse, therefore, people taking treatment, and their treatment assistants, are positioned as effective treatment citizens alongside medical professionals, forming contingent alliances with medical discourse, negotiating with it, disseminating this negotiated treatment knowledge socially and negotiating with it further in the process (Robins, 2008). This engagement is borrowed for public discourse, as it was in developing-world epidemics, from its earlier activist and community incarnations (Davis et al., 2006; Epstein, 1996). In the Western Cape, this discourse was at least partly effective in practice. The drive towards treatment literacy in advance of scaleup set up an important HIV sociality of people throughout the province, discussing ART in families and friendship networks as well as CBOs and NGOs. This sociality appeared in the early-2000s concern of many people living around the demonstration and initial scaleup sites to 'speak out' about their status, and how one can live with and be treated for HIV as an illness, not as a sign of social or spiritual transgression (Squire, 2007). The sociality of scaleup itself, institutionalised in the decentred structure of local clinics' implementation strategies, allowed patients' groups and CBOs input into guidelines for starting and supporting treatment. These discussions migrated outward into broader family, friendship and community socialities. Such a socialised treatment citizenship technology seems now to extend across the province, and may be another factor contributing to the Western Cape's high HIV test rates, and the rise in sexual debut age in the province (Flisher et al., 2006) – something often said to be associated with the plateauing of other high-prevalence epidemics (Epstein, 2006).

Treatment citizenship could be seen as a kind of 'capacity building'. Campbell is rightly sceptical about this process, describing it as fatally self-undermining. Generally, efforts at building treatment citizenship technologies, or Campbell's broader category of HIV competence, try to correct resource inequities by transferring resources defined by those that have them, who also decide how they shall be transferred and when they have been successfully moved over. Such programmes' understanding of power differences is undercut by their re-performance of these differences precisely while combating them. The contested nature of politics (Mouffe, 2005) is acknowledged in analysis, erased in implementation. In the case of the Western Cape scaleup however, the technology of treatment citizenship was to a large extent defined, appropriated and developed by the people requiring it.

Treatment citizenship is not equivalent to HIV citizenship in general, but its technology may build that broader formation. We have seen how the province's prevalent forms of treatment citizenship seem associated with high levels of HIV testing, and changes in sexual relationship patterns. In addition, Western Cape treatment citizenship generated, and continues to support, jointly developed campaigns by medical professionals, NGOs and CBOs, for cheap access to key license-protected drugs; but also NGOs' and CBOs' development of support services, for instance around gender violence. CBOs' involvement in treatment education has led to stronger prevention and education programmes, an integration of great concern to people of all statuses in South Africa. With the help of a supportive doctor, Western Cape women enrolled in PMTCT programmes began educating other pregnant positive women, a commitment now formalised in 'Mothers2mothers2B' groups which have spread across South Africa and other southern African countries (http://www.m2m.org/). ART support groups, concentrated at the beginning of treatment, have spun off income generation projects. People 'speaking out' about HIV as a treatable, liveable-with illness, promote dialogue not just about HIV status and treatment, but also about HIV's nature, prevention, and implications for the nation and the future (Daniel and Squire, 2009).

Even in talking of their treatment 'rights' as citizens, people living with HIV in the Western Cape assert 'rights' in ways that are not restricted to treatment or health citizenship exclusively, but that do not either become generalised assertions of 'human' rights (Robins, 2008). Between 2001 and 2004, for example, Squire's interviewees articulated 'rights' particularly and transitively in relation to HIV's impact in different fields, specifying entitlements to goods in health, social, employment and education fields. HIV positive people demanded treatment, but also food for their children once PTMCT programmes – which provide infant formula – had been completed, and food for themselves to promote the success of ART (an issue of which scaleup programme directors were well aware – see Abdullah, 2004). They asked for funeral grants for family members who died of HIV, and for flexible disability grants, since even with ART, continuous paid work can be problematic for HIV positive people, assuming they can get such work. They wanted training that would enable them to work in areas suitable for chronically ill people. This specificity about who has rights, and to what, clarifies convergences and distinctions between HIV positive and other citizens, that is, their equivalent identities (Mouffe, 2005), while also defining contemporary HIV citizenship in ways that go beyond treatment citizenship. The technology of HIV citizenship built up through the roll-out can then be summarised as a pragmatic citizenship, equivalent with but not identical to the citizenship of the non-HIV affected, that lays out commonalities with other citizens, while still marking the important particularities of the condition.

In addition, people living with or alongside the demonstration projects and scaleup have developed HIV citizenship as a moral formation. They describe how to live well as HIV positive citizens in ways that speak back to HIV's social and religious pathologisation, and that closely match broader South African understandings of good conduct and appropriate ways of living. They adumbrate a pragmatic 'somatic ethics' (Rose, 2007: 252) involving care of the self through cleanliness, diet and exercise; care of others – children, partners and neighbours; cooking and cleaning; paid work when possible; and a social commitment to speaking and acting truthfully and ethically – in this case, about HIV. These formulations of care of self and others within HIV citizenship technology relate to the principle of *ubuntu*, the humanity inherent in living through and for others, mentioned by some of Squire's (2007) interviewees and a frequent point of cultural and political reference in South Africa. Interviewees emphasised that a person living with HIV was 'still' a person and not an animal, and must be socially recognised as such, despite their specific characteristics and requirements. Such formulations embed politically equivalent HIV citizenship in ethical but still pragmatic considerations about how to live well in specific contexts, including that of HIV.

We have suggested that the Western Cape ART scaleup can be analysed as working through a triad of administrative, partnership and citizenship technologies, built up from near-zero in some places and cases, to high and largely self-sustaining levels. The scaleup technologies were not necessarily or exactly connected with people's development of a wider HIV citizenship; they had some independent fields of action. However it is clear that they contributed to the constitution of this broader HIV citizenship within the province. These technologies can be worked with in other contexts, but crucial to their effectiveness has been their recognition of factors that must be addressed locally. Such particularity, instantiated in the scaleup's commitment to neighbourhood-developed strategies, renders the technologies resistant to exact translation.

The technologies also present substantial problems of contemporary and future implementation, derived from their own heterogeneities and contradictions, as well as from those that appear in their relation with other medical, social and political technologies.

The limits of scaleup technologies

Throughout the scaleup, its technologies have encountered a number of resistances, some of which are likely to persist and strengthen. The scaleup has not made HIV citizens of the 20,000 people estimated to be HIV positive and to need treatment, who are not accessing it. Partial explanations for this may lie, as mentioned earlier, in the limitations of the programme's administrative technology, particularly in health service resources reaching their limits. In addition to the general programme, the health department is now targeting the specific local problematics of HIV in relation to older men, schoolchildren, sex workers and truck drivers. The scaleup may also have encountered a geographic limit in reaching people who can access clinics by walking or by car; many rural settlements are not served by roads. As people live longer, the complications of long-term ART use become more common, more people progress to ART, increasing numbers move onto expensive second- and third-line drug regimes and incidence remains high, problems will multiply. Men, who have little contact with South

African health services, are consistently under-represented in treatment at 30% of the total – though more women are HIV positive (Boulle et al., 2008). Women continue to face gendered stigmatisation and disclosure difficulties (Ratele and Shefer, 2002; Rohleder and Gibson, 2006). HIV's dramatic impact at diagnosis and its stigmatisation persists, in South Africa and globally (Flowers, this volume; Stevens and Hildebrandt, 2006). Acknowledging the condition, disclosing (Flowers, this volume) embarking on lifelong medication, and dealing with side effects and HIV's ongoing medical uncertainties (Davis, this volume; Olley et al., 2005) continue to be difficult. New prevention issues arise for those taking ARTs or simply having sex in the ART era, particularly for women who are now formulating their AIDS-era sexualities in new ways. Younger people particularly are becoming accustomed to, even bored with HIV, as this high-prevalence epidemic moves into a second decade of public awareness and action.

All these characteristics suggest the importance of 'psychosocial' factors to which, as mentioned earlier, medical, NGO and CBO partnership technology in the scaleup have not yet made full responses. Given the newness, high prevalence, particularity and fluidity of this epidemic, an expectation that neighbourhoods and communities could develop their own fully adequate and sustainable support mechanisms to cover all these areas of the 'psychosocial' out of ART partnership technologies, would be over-optimistic. The 'psychosocial' itself may need redefinition within ART technologies (Wilbraham, this volume). Moreover, while the scaleup programme certainly acknowledges the multiple dimensions of what we have called 'treatment citizenship', that citizenship's overtly political and educative elements have been privileged. Its more diffuse sociality is harder to describe, let alone encourage; and it is always under challenge. For though everyone in South Africa is in some way 'living with' HIV, the 'equivalence' between different citizens – between HIV positive women and men, the positive well and the symptomatic, the infected and the affected, parents and their children – is approximate, changing and contested.

A further criticism addresses the scaleup's medical focus. Does this focus inevitably 'medicalise' HIV citizenship? Treatment-oriented responses to the pandemic are frequently accused of reducing people's relations with HIV to that of patients and research subjects' relations to disease and virus. This accusation also applies to recent treatment-oriented prevention discourse that, instead of focusing on personal and social action, promotes early (Granich et al., 2009) or prophylactic (Rosengarten, this volume) ART. Microbicides and circumcision, ART post-sexual assault, even condoms and clean needles, can also be conceptualised as medicalisations of prevention. Such criticisms often link to broader condemnations of subjects' and whole economies' co-option by pharma-capital, and of developing countries' surveillance by international NGOs such as the WHO. However, to equate treatment activism, at for instance the Western Cape neighbourhood or local government level, with international treatment capitalism and post-colonial regulation, seems patronisingly over-simplifying. There is, too, considerable heterogeneity within the biopolitics of both international NGOs and pharmacological companies, which are also not the least socially responsible or responsive corporate sector. South Africa is in addition, like many other sub-Saharan African countries, trying to expand its own 'small pharma' production of ART drugs, a development that, like developing countries' production of generics, complicates biocapital analysis.

The 'medicalisation' critique of treatment scaleup is most aptly countered in the Western Cape case by the programme's actualities. Even when the scaleup's non-medical partners developed medical expertise, they did not become medical*ised* citizens wholly co-opted by western medical discourse and practice. Most people taking ART for instance also use traditional and complementary approaches they think appropriate, often in consultation with their doctors, as indeed happens across developing- and developed-world HIV epidemics and in developing-world health care in general. While patients have high treatment literacy and commitment, they are not generally strongly identified with medical expertise. Their relations with their doctors tend to be relatively conventional partnerships, with patient and practitioner roles clearly separated. More importantly, the *non-medical* technologies that we have described were key to scaleup's success. Administrative and partnership technologies were formulated and implemented with relative autonomy from the medical technologies of ART. Even treatment citizenship, the technology most focussed on medicine, configured health information in terms of activism and social dialogue, and had important associations with broader forms of HIV citizenship.

Conclusion

How will the Western Cape programme's scaleup technologies fare in the future? The plan is for double enrolment yearly for the next five years, particularly focusing on under-represented men. As more patients stay on therapy, more will move to expensive second-line drugs. The number of people requiring treatment will continue to rise well into the next decade and beyond, if numbers of new cases do not fall (Western Cape Department of Health, 2006). The resourcing of such extensive treatment, even given generic provision and domestic manufacture, will be a growing concern. The psychological, social and political consequences for large fractions of the population living long-term with difficult medical treatment are hard to predict. Achmat and Simcock (2007) are optimistic about the ameliorative effects of long-term treatment combined with prevention, education and community mobilisation – the wider HIV citizenship technologies discussed above. Draper et al. (2007) call for large-scale and thoroughgoing initiatives that do not look qualitatively different from those currently operating. The citizenship, administrative and partnership strategies discussed here, may, despite their limitations, be able to address at least some of the future conditions of this epidemic, and perhaps of others.

References

Abdullah, F. (2004) 'The complexity of implementing antirretroviral therapy in the Western Cape province of South Africa', in M. Heyward (ed.) *From disaster to development? HIV and AIDS in Southern Africa, Development Update* 5, 3, 245–64.

—— (2006) 'Lessons from the field; ART scaleup in South Africa. XVIth International AIDS Conference, Toronto.

Abdullah, F., Bock, P., Osler, M. and Boulle, A. (2006) 'Clinical outcomes in ART scaleup, Western Cape Province of South Africa', XVIth International AIDS Conference, Toronto.

Achmat, Z. and Simcock, J. (2007) 'Combining prevention, treatment and care: lessons from South Africa', *AIDS*, 21, Suppl. 4, S11–S20.

Beresford, B. (2004) 'Pioneering treatment access in a rural area of South Africa', in M. Heyward (ed.) *From disaster to development? HIV and AIDS in Southern Africa, Development Update*, 5, 3, 277–92.

Boulle, A., Bock, P., Osler, M., Cohen, K., Channing, L., Hildebrand, K., Mothibi, E., Zweigenthal, V., Slingers, N., Cloete, K. and Abdullah, F. (2008) 'Antiretroviral therapy and early mortality in South Africa', *WHO Bulletin*, 86, 678–87.

Campbell, C. (2003) *Letting them die?* (Oxford: James Currey).

Campbell, C., Nair, Y., Maimane, S. and Sibiya, Z. (2007) 'Building contexts that support effective community responses to HIV/AIDS', *American Journal of Community Psychology*, 39, 3–4, 347–63.

Chesney, M. and Smith, A. (1999) 'Critical delays in HIV testing and care: the potential role of stigma', *American Behavioural Scientist*, 42, 1162–74.

Coetzee, D., Hildebrand, K., Boulle, A., Maartens, G., Louis, F., Labatala, V., Reuter, H., Ntwana, N. and Goemaere, E. (2004) 'Outcomes after two years of providing antiretroviral treatment in Khayelitsha, South Africa', *AIDS*, 18, 887–95.

Daniel, L. and Squire, C. (2009) 'Experiences of people living with HIV', in P. Rohleder, L. Swartz, S. Kalichman and L. Simbayi (eds) *HIV/AIDS in South Africa 25 years on* (New York: Springer).

Davis, M., Frankis, J. and Flowers, P. (2006) 'Uncertainty and technological horizon in qualitative interviews about HIV treatment', *Health*, 10, 3, 323–44.

Draper, B., Pienaar, D., Parker, W. and Rehle, T. (2007 'Recommendations for policy in the Western Cape Province for the prevention of major infectious Diseases, including HIV/AIDS and tuberculosis' (Cape Town: Western Cape Department of Health).

Cape Town: Provincial Government of the Western Cape (2006). 'The Western Cape Antiretroviral Programme: Monitoring Report', http://web.uct.ac.za/depts/epi/artrollout/files/Artmonitoringreport_wc_062006.pdf, 12 July 2008.

Epstein, H. (2006) *The invisible cure* (New York: Farrar, Straus and Giroux).

Epstein, S. (1996) *Impure science: AIDS, activism and the politics of knowledge* (Los Angeles, CA: University of California Press).

Flisher, A., Matthews, C., Mukoma, W. and Lombard, C. (2006) 'Secular trends in risk behaviour of Cape Town Grade 8 students', *South African Medical Journal*, 99, 9, part 2, 982–7, September.

Flowers, P., Davis, M., Hart, G., Rosengarten, M., Frankis, J. and Imrie, J. (2006) 'Diagnosis and stigma and identity amongst HIV positive Black Africans living in the UK', *Psychology and Health*, 21, 1, 109–22.

Foucault, M. (1980) *History of sexuality volume 1* (London: Allen Lane).

Freire, P. (1973). *Education for critical consciousness* (New York: Continuum).

Granich, R., Gilks, C., Dye, C., De Cock, K. and Williams, B. (2009) 'Universal voluntary HIV testing with immediate antiretroviral therapy as a strategy for elimination of HIV transmission: a mathematical model', *Lancet*, 373, 9657, 48–57.

Heywood, M. (2004) 'Editor's preface', in M. Heywood (ed.) *From disaster to development? HIV and AIDS in Southern Africa, Development Update*, 5, 3, 3–16.

Hutchinson, P. and Mahlalela, X. (2006) 'Utilisation of voluntary counselling and testing services in the Eastern Cape, South Africa', *AIDS Care*, 18, 5, 446–55.

Infectious Disease Epidemiology Unit UCT/Department of Health (2006) *Models of care for antiretroviral service delivery* (Cape Town: Western Cape Department of Health).

Jackson, D., Chopra, M., Doherty, T., Colvin, M., Levin, J., Willumsen, J., Goga, A. and Moodley, P. for the Good Start Study Group (2007) 'Operational effectiveness and 36-week HIV-free survival in the South African programme to prevent mother-to-child transmission of HIV-1', *AIDS*, 21, 509–16.

Jewkes, R. (2009) 'HIV and women', in P. Rohleder, L. Swartz, S. Kalichman and L. Simbayi (eds) *HIV/AIDS in South Africa 25 years on* (New York: Springer).

Mbali, M. (2005) 'The Treatment Action Campaign and the history of rights based patient-driven HIV/AIDS activism in South Africa', *Centre for Civil Society Research Report*, 29, 1–23.

Moodley, D., Moodley, J., Coovadia, H., Gray, G., McIntyre, J., Hofmyer, J., Nikodem, C., Hall, D., Gigliotti, M., Robinson, P., Boshoff, L., and Sullivan, J. (2003) 'A multi-center randomized controlled trial of nevirapine versus a combination of zidovudine and lamivudine to reduce intrapartum and early postpartum mother-to-child transmission of human immunodeficiency virus type 1', *Journal of Infectious Diseases*, 187, 725–35.

Mouffe, C. (2005) *The return of the political* (London: Verso).

Naimak, T. (2006) 'Antiretroviral treatment in the Western Cape', CSSR Working Paper 161, http:///www.cssr.ac.za/index/htm, 12 July 2008.

Olley, B., Zeier, M., Seedat, S. and Stein, D. (2005) 'Post-traumatic stress disorder among recently diagnosed patients with HIV/AIDS in South Africa', *AIDS Care*, 17, 5, 550–7.

Rabinow, P. (1996) *Essays on the anthropology of reason* (Princeton: Princeton University Press).

Ratele, K. and Shefer, T. (2002) 'Stigma in the social construction of sexually transmitted diseases', in D. Hook and G. Eagle (eds) *Psychopathology and social prejudice* (Cape Town: University of Cape Town Press).

Republic of South Africa (2008) 'Progress report on the declaration of commitment on HIV/AIDS', http://data.unaids.org/pub/Report/2008/south_africa_2008_country_progress_report_en.pdf, 12 July 2008.

Robins, S. (2008) *From revolution to rights in South Africa* (Durban: UKZN Press).

Rofes, E. (1998) *Dry bones breathe* (New York: Harrington Park Press).

Rohleder, P. and Gibson, K. (2006). '"We are not fresh": HIV-positive women talk of their experience of living with their spoiled identity', *South African Journal of Psychology*, 36, 1, 25–44.

Rose, N. (2007) *The politics of life itself* (Princeton, NJ: Princeton University Press).

Skogmar, S., Shkaeley, D., Lam, M., Daniell, J., Andersson, R., Tshandu, N., Odón, A., Roberts, S. and Venter, F. (2006) 'Effects of antiretroviral treatment and counselling on disclosure of HIV serostatus in Johannesburg, South Africa', *AIDS Care*, 18, 7, 725–30.

Squire, C. (2007) *HIV in South Africa*, London: Routledge.

Stevens P. and Hildebrandt, E. (2006) 'Life changing words: women's responses to being diagnosed with HIV infection', *Advances in Nursing Science*, 29, 3, 207–21.

Sunder, K., (2006) *Biocapital* (Durham, NC: Duke University Press).

UNAIDS (2008) 'AIDS epidemic update', http://www.unaids.org/en/HIV_data/epi2008/default.asp, 4 March 2009.

Uys, P. (2008) 'Western Cape Health Budget 2008/9', http://www.capegateway.gov.za/other/2008/5/wc_health_budget_speech_2008.pdf, 2 May 2009.

Western Cape Department of Health (2006) 'The Western Cape antiretroviral programme monitoring report', http://www.capegateway.gov.za/eng/pubs/reports_research/W/157844, 12 July 2008.

Wolfe, W., Weiser, S., Leiter, K., Steward, W., Percy-de Korte, F., Phaladze, N., Iacopino, V. and Heisler, M. (2008) 'The impact of universal access to antiretroviral therapy on HIV stigma in Botswana, *American Journal of Public Health*, 98, 10, 1865–71.

World Health Organization (2003) *Antiretroviral treatment in primary health care: experience of the Khayelitsha programme in South Africa* (Geneva: World Health Organisation) http://www.who.int/hiv/pub/prev_care/en/South_Africa_E.pdf, 4 March 2009.

—— (2006) *Progress on global access to HIV antiretroviral therapy* (Geneva: World Health Organization), http://www.who.int/hiv/progressreport2006_en.pdf, 12 July 2008.
—— (2009) *Towards universal access: scaling up priority HIV/AIDS interventions in the health sector: progress report* (Geneva: World Health Organization), http://www.who.int/hiv/pub/2009progressreport/en/print.html , 30 September 2009.

4

Integrating HIV Treatment and Prevention: Shifts in Community-based Organising and Biopolitics in the Canadian Context

Eric Mykhalovskiy

Introduction

Important changes are underway in how the relationship between HIV prevention and treatment is understood and enacted in global AIDS work. Historically, prevention and treatment have been configured as distinct strategies for responding to HIV infection. Rooted in the rationality and techniques of public health, HIV prevention has focused on securing the health of the 'general population'. By contrast, antiretroviral therapy (ART), a central technology of biomedicine, has sought to restore individual, damaged human bodies. Health care, frontline, policy and research responses to HIV have often cleaved along recognised distinctions between the forms of reason, technologies, objectives and targets of public health and biomedicine.

Recent efforts to 'roll out' HIV treatment in the global South coupled with scientific research on the potential value of ART for preventing the sexual transmission of HIV have challenged the specificity of HIV prevention and treatment. Rather than emphasising their distinctiveness, current thinking calls for ways of linking or connecting treatment with prevention. This has been materialised in a popular and widespread discourse of 'integration'. Much of the discussion about integrating HIV treatment and prevention has been carried forward through policy and/or epidemiological research and writing. In this chapter, by contrast, I draw attention to the play of integration discourse in the politics of community-based AIDS organizing in Canada.

Canada is a country with a vast geography, but a relatively small population of 33 million (Statistics Canada, 2009). HIV prevalence in Canada is low with an estimated 58,000 persons living with HIV (including AIDS) at the end of 2005 (Public Health Agency of Canada, 2007). Canada's

HIV epidemic is also regionally and demographically concentrated with the country's four most populous provinces (Ontario, Quebec, British Columbia and Alberta) accounting for over 95% of reported HIV and AIDS diagnoses (Public Health Agency of Canada, 2007). 'Men who have sex with men' make up 51% of prevalent infections, followed by injection drug users at 17% of total cases (Public Health Agency of Canada, 2007). From the outset of the epidemic in Canada, community-based AIDS organisations have played a vital role in the frontline response to HIV and in lobbying for improved government response to the epidemic. This chapter focuses on the activities of one such organisation, the Canadian AIDS Treatment Information Exchange (CATIE).

In developing my analysis I have been inspired by Flyvbjerg's vision of a 'social science that matters' (2001). Flyvbjerg argues that the project of a social science built through analogy with the natural sciences and the pursuit of predictive or general explanatory theory is ill-fated. The alternative he recommends is to recuperate social science by emphasising its relationship to forms of practical knowledge of the sort suggested by Aristotle's notion of phronesis. By centring social science in a reinterpretation of phronesis that more fully incorporates questions of power, Flyvbjerg encourages a social science that aims at a reflexive knowledge for social practice. Rather than valuing a scientific knowledge of and for the general, social scientists would commit to a knowledge of the particular case – to a context-specific, concrete knowledge that addresses issues of value and power.

Flyvbjerg's emphasis on context-dependent knowledge offers a welcome alternative to the established forms of discussion of integration found in the academic literature. Epidemiological and policy-based analyses of integrating HIV treatment and prevention orient to questions of global pandemic management and privilege high levels of abstraction. They also tend to lionise integration as a complementary union of treatment and prevention and advocate for it as universal policy and programme objective.

By contrast, my discussion of integration privileges the concrete and local. I do not advocate for integration, nor is my analysis organised by the policy object of global HIV pandemic management. Instead, my interest is to explore how integration discourse is understood and realised in the context of everyday community-based AIDS work and with what implications. My discussion treats CATIE as a case study from which to consider how integration is made meaningful within the trajectory of a given organisation's history, how it is brought into being through concrete work activities and what challenges it presents, given a particular configuration of community-based HIV treatment politics.

To develop my analysis, I draw on almost 20 years of involvement with CATIE as a former staff member, board director and volunteer. I also make use of a total of 16 semi-structured qualitative interviews conducted with CATIE staff, representatives from funding agencies and participants involved in a CATIE initiative focused on integration. I also rely on multiple informal conversations with CATIE staff and AIDS activists in Toronto, my participation in the Toronto-based activist groups AIDS ACTION NOW! and the Ontario Working Group on Criminal Law and HIV Exposure as well as on a reading of the established literature on integration.

The chapter begins with a short critical review of the literature on integrating HIV treatment and prevention. I argue that the literature advances a way of thinking about integration that emphasises the complementarity of treatment and prevention. I then turn to a discussion of the formative politics of CATIE. I argue that the establishment of CATIE was informed by activist thought that sharply distinguished between the political rationalities of HIV prevention and treatment. This distinction was central to a social movement politics, constitutive of CATIE, that associated HIV, a politics of health and life, and the pursuit of biomedical treatment access, with lasting implications for the organisation. Next, the chapter explores how CATIE has responded to integration. Drawing on multiple examples I suggest that the primary response has been one of organisational accommodation. CATIE has used integration as an organisational solution to a number of problems associated with its established programmatic orientation to treatment information. I note, however, that organisational accommodation has its limits. Two developments associated with integration – positive prevention and biomedical prevention – resurface tensions between prevention and a treatment-centred politics of health connected with PHAs. At the same time they point to ways of reimagining HIV treatment as an object of biopolitics that centre on the question of responsibility for HIV transmission.

A short history of integration discourse

The integration of HIV treatment and prevention has recently emerged as an important element of global HIV/AIDS response. It is informed by and circulates throughout multiple, intersecting sites of biomedical, epidemiological, policy, public health and community-based research and practice. Integration discourse is heterogeneous, its articulation inflected with the organisational priorities and positionings of its interlocutors, including, for example the characteristic development discourse of UNAIDS and a unique moral representation of AIDS response characteristic of 'Partners in Health', an initiative affiliated with the Harvard School of Public Health and focused on providing primary health care in less-developed countries, particularly Haiti. My concern here is not to explore these and related differences of nuance and framing that surface across the sites of articulation of integration. Rather, my concern is to emphasise how integration coheres as a discourse focused on pandemic management that emphasises the putative complementarity of HIV treatment and prevention initiatives.

An important formative expression of integration discourse can be found in the research of physician and anthropologist Paul Farmer. Farmer has written about integration with colleagues working out of Partners in Health (Farmer, 2003; Farmer et al. (2006 [1992]); Koenig, Leandre and Farmer, 2004). Farmer positions integration as a corrective to arguments that force a choice between treatment or prevention in responding to the HIV pandemic in less developed countries. He critiques the historical privileging of prevention, noting that it is 'time to turn ... attention to the more than 30 million individuals already living with HIV' (Farmer et al., 2001: 404). He and his colleagues further argue that effective delivery of HIV care in resource-poor settings is not only feasible, but also benefits HIV prevention. A commonly cited finding of their research is that the introduction of ART by village health care workers in Haiti enhanced voluntary counselling and HIV antibody testing (Mukherjee and Eustache, 2007; Walton, Farmer, Lambert et al., 2004). Overall, they represent HIV care and prevention not as mutually exclusive alternatives, but as complementary resources that go hand in hand in responding to the HIV pandemic.

Integration has also been popularised in a more general, policy-oriented literature on the global management of the HIV pandemic. The central interlocutors have been public health researchers as well representatives from international and non-governmental organisations such as WHO, the Global Fund to Fight AIDS, Tuberculosis and Malaria, the Bill and Melinda Gates Foundation and the Joint United Nations Programme on HIV/AIDS (Global HIV Prevention Working Group, 2004; Salomon et al., 2005; Schwartländer et al., 2006). The literature is organised primarily as a reflection on the WHO/UNAIDS '3 by 5' programme to increase access to ART in developing countries.[1]

While the literature recognises potential tensions between treatment and prevention, it nevertheless presents integration as a central dimension of future global HIV pandemic management. One line of argument draws on epidemiological reasoning and a calculus of health outcomes to argue in favour of integrating HIV treatment and prevention. For example,

Salomon et al. (2005) project that 50% more new infections and twice as many deaths are prevented with an integrated response as compared to the use of prevention alone. They argue that HIV prevention can make treatment affordable, while 'treatment can make prevention more effective' (2005: 55). Once again neither approach alone is understood to offer a successful global response to HIV. Only when they are integrated can 'sustained progress in the global fight against HIV/AIDS' be made (2005: 50).

Another line of argument uses the convention of 'lessons learned' from the 3 by 5 initiative to bolster the case for integration. Schwartländer, Grubb and Perriëns (2006) argue that widespread access to treatments has helped to de-stigmatise HIV and has enhanced possibilities for open communication about HIV prevention. They describe the choice between treatment or prevention as a 'false dichotomy', that must be overcome in order to 'finally turn the epidemic around' (2006: 545). Gayle and Lange (2004) and Shodell (2006) similarly argue that while prevention was not an explicit part of '3 by 5', treatment roll-out nevertheless made visible important synergies between treatment and prevention. For example, they note that as treatments were distributed, people were drawn into health care settings where HIV prevention messages were enhanced. Like Farmer and colleagues, they note that HIV testing and counselling were popularised as expanded treatment access created opportunities for developing HIV prevention strategies that drew on the involvement of people living with HIV (PLHIV). Observations of this sort are used in the literature to support a call for a new strategic direction in pandemic management that will realise the putative complementarity of treatment and prevention. The vision is one in which 'false dichotomies' are abandoned in favour of a 'carefully coordinated' (Gayle and Lange, 2006: 6) and 'balanced and comprehensive approach' (Shodell, 2006: 1) to simultaneous scale up of prevention and treatment (Global HIV Prevention Working Group, 2004).

Finally, the growing significance of integration discourse in global AIDS work is suggested by its widespread presence at the 2006 International AIDS Conference held in Toronto, Canada. Integration approached the status of 'mantra' in Toronto, its central elements expressed by multiple conference participants including those speaking at the session 'Getting the balance right: Integrating HIV prevention and treatment programming.' Claims that 'we cannot treat our way out of this epidemic' (De Cock, 2006), that 'there can be no prevention without treatment and no treatment without prevention' (Hassan, 2006), that the choice between treatment or prevention is a 'false dichotomy' (Simao, 2006) and that treatment and prevention are a 'seamless continuum' (Binder, 2006) circulated widely throughout the conference. They helped organise the peculiar moral force of integration discourse at the conference in which abstract claims about complementarity were used to mark a break between a sad past of competitive relations between treatment and prevention and a hopeful future of collaboration and balance.[2]

It is important to recognise that integration discourse is not only about the forms of complementarity of treatment and prevention emphasised at the 2006 International AIDS Conference and developed in the literature. The established discourse on integration accommodates tension in the relationship between treatment and prevention. As suggested above, the history of global management is typically represented as one of ongoing imbalance between prevention and treatment with early years marked by an overemphasis on prevention followed by an over-focus on treatments in the wake of the 3 by 5 initiative. Thus, while integration discourse may encourage an understanding of treatment and prevention as seamless, the very need to argue the case so strongly suggests how that seamlessness is always an active, ongoing and potentially fragile achievement.

To sum up, in the context of HIV, integration coordinates a general discourse of pandemic management that circulates widely across sites of HIV response globally. Integration discourse is marked most prominently by its promotion of integration as a preferred response to stemming the tide of HIV infection. With the exception of discussions of attempts to link treatment and prevention in clinical settings in less-developed countries, integration is treated at fairly highly levels of abstraction. Integration is at risk of being reduced to a type of mantra or truism of global AIDS work. To mitigate this, accounts of integration are needed that escape the celebration of complementarity and that explore actual efforts to link treatment and prevention in locally situated organisational work.

The case study – CATIE

CATIE was established in 1990 in Toronto, Canada, as a community-based organisation committed to producing and distributing treatment information for people living with HIV and AIDS, their health care providers, and others who support them. Antinomies associated with the historical organisational focus of CATIE – information on biomedical treatments for HIV infection – make it an interesting site for exploring the implications of integration for community-based AIDS organising. So too does a recent extension of the organisation's mandate to include the support of HIV prevention efforts through the exchange and distribution of HIV prevention information. Since 2008, CATIE has refashioned its identity from an organisation oriented exclusively to

HIV treatment information to one now concerned with treatment *and* prevention.

CATIE grew out of a Toronto-based activist organisation called AIDS ACTION NOW! (AAN!) which was founded in 1988. The history and activities of AAN! are similar to those of AIDS activist organisations established in the early years of the epidemic in the US, such as ACT UP New York. Like ACT UP New York, AAN! was established primarily by activists from the gay rights movement, many of whom were PLHIV, who had come together over concerns related to problems with medical care, access to treatments and the state of clinical trials research. The significance of the ACT UP network for challenging the pharmaceutical industry and intervening in the conduct of HIV-related clinical trials research has been duly noted (Epstein 1996; Epstein 2000; Smith and Siplon, 2006). Like ACT UP New York, AAN! targeted pharmaceutical science in its political work, notably compelling authorities to terminate an unethical pentamidine trial in 1989 and, the same year, forcing the compassionate release of ddI. Unlike ACT UP, however, the central focus of AAN!'s activist work was the state, at both federal and provincial levels. The US notoriously lacks a system of public health insurance. In Canada, the state has played a much more significant role in the organisation of health care, financing through medicare, those 'medically necessary services' provided by physicians or delivered in hospitals.[3] The greater expectation for state involvement in health care in Canada shaped AAN!'s targeting of the state for its inaction in the early years of the epidemic in Canada.

The critique of government response to HIV in Canada developed by AAN! was central to the formation of CATIE. AAN! sharply distinguished between the political projects associated with HIV treatment and prevention. In the late 1980s and early 1990s, prominent AAN! member and sociologist George Smith (1990) argued convincingly that the response to HIV/AIDS in Canada was overwhelmingly shaped by the rationalities and technologies of public health. This early public health framing of HIV represented a site of contestation for AAN! members who argued for an alternative representation of HIV as a clinical problem and health concern for those already living with HIV and AIDS (Smith, 1990).

Smith argued that while HIV infection presented innumerable clinical challenges, state authorities were oriented only to preventing infectious disease transmission. They viewed HIV as an infectious disease threat, one that could have devastating effects at the population level if not contained. As such, their principal concern was to limit or stop the spread of infection, rather than facilitate a coordinated response to the clinical needs of those already infected with HIV. In Smith's analysis the state basically lacked an effective organisational mechanism for managing the treatment response required of an emerging infectious disease like HIV/AIDS. The problematisation of HIV as a clinical phenomenon was the preserve of the medical profession which, at the time, viewed HIV as a little more than a terminal illness. Unaccustomed to intervening in the clinical content of biomedicine and lacking an active apparatus for testing new treatments or making experimental treatments readily available, state response to HIV became firmly lodged in a logic of prevention, while early biomedical response to HIV in Canada rarely surpassed palliation (Smith, 1995).

The position developed by Smith and AAN! underscored how the health needs of people already infected with HIV were external to the dominant forms of HIV epidemic management in Canada. An anecdote told by Tim McCaskell, a co-chair of AAN! who helped organise the activist storming of the main stage at the International AIDS Conference in Montreal in 1989, captures the forms of public health reasoning that he, Smith and others sought to confront at the time. In McCaskell's account, Alistair Clayton, then director of Canada's Federal Centre for AIDS remarked during the Montreal conference that treatments for HIV were not needed because once prevention efforts stopped the spread of HIV, the reservoir of infection would die off.[4]

AAN! helped establish a political direction for CATIE that was based on an understanding of an antagonistic relationship between treatment and prevention and that emphasised a very different relationship of the two to the health needs of PLHIV. Local AIDS activists, particularly those living with HIV, viewed prevention as irrelevant if not contrary to their interests. Public health technologies of prevention, particularly strategies of containment and the delineation of risk groups, were understood as efforts that went toward protecting the health of the 'general population', not to responding to the immediate health crisis faced by those living with HIV or AIDS. From the standpoint of people living with HIV and AIDS, what was required at the time was political and organisational work that intervened in the management of the HIV epidemic to make biomedical treatments a reality for HIV+ people. While the route of argument took a different path, like organisations such as ACT UP New York, AAN! formulated a biopolitics centred on the object of medical treatment. It aligned the interests of an emerging social movement of people living with HIV and AIDS and a politics of life and health that sought to stimulate the production of and increase in social access to biomedical treatment.

CATIE was conceived as a contribution to that politics. The organisation began as a volunteer committee of AAN!, but formalised its operations when I was hired as its first staff member through funding from the

Ontario Trillium Foundation in 1990. CATIE quickly became successful in securing funding for its work and evolved organisationally along the lines of other local community-based AIDS organisations (Cain, 2002), with the exception that its governing board for many years comprised local AIDS activists. An important turning point occurred in the mid-1990s when CATIE received funding to extend its operations to a national level.

CATIE offers an interesting example of how HIV treatments operate as boundary- and institution-making technologies (Biehl, 2008). Historically, CATIE distinguished itself from other Canadian community-based AIDS organisations through its emphasis on HIV treatment. In the North American context, during its early years, CATIE was part of a small group of initiatives centred on providing community-based HIV treatment information that included, for example, Philadelphia's Critical Path AIDS Project, *AIDS Treatment News*, then based in San Francisco, and *Treatment Issues*, published by The Gay Men's Health Crisis in New York. Whereas other community-based AIDS organisations in Canada provided counselling, support and prevention services, CATIE prided itself as the country's only community-based organisation focused solely on providing and distributing HIV treatment information. CATIE carried forward its foundational politics and built an organisational identity by sidestepping the realm of prevention and by establishing the distribution of treatment information as a primary community-based strategy for meeting the health needs of PLHIV.

This political project has not been without its tensions and ambiguities. For one thing, CATIE's focus on clinically oriented information has meant the support of a notion of health centred on the individual body and oriented to its restoration through clinical means of a primarily biomedical sort. The provision of information about the social determinants of health has been less well-developed. In mediating between formal health information and lay health knowledge, CATIE embraces sources of alternative health information and also circulates people's experiential knowledge about HIV and taking treatments (Mykhalovskiy, 2008). However, the primary dynamics of its knowledge mediation involve simplifying complex biomedical information for audiences of PLHIV.

Tensions also surface around CATIE's chosen object: health information. These centre on questions about what can be taken to be its most useful form and content as well as the extent of people's interest in health information and the social contours of its potential to improve the health of people living with HIV and AIDS. While CATIE operates a 1-800 treatment enquiry service, historically, it has privileged text-based forms of health information. CATIE has produced a range of important publications including *TreatmentUpdate, Managing Your Health, The Positive Side* and numerous web-based treatment resources (for details, see www.catie.ca).

Instrumentalising health information as printed text is often associated with the trope of rational decision making and its many assumptions about the knower of health information and the nature of his or her healthwork. The imagined user is typically middle-class, accustomed to orienting to texts as meaningful resources in daily life and to using biomedical information to inform personal health choices and decisions. Widespread research on the experience of living with HIV as well as other chronic illnesses shows just how far people's healthwork exceeds the limits of a rational engagement with text-based health information (Ferzacca, 2000; McCoy, 2005; Mykhalovskiy, McCoy and Breaslier, 2004; Persson, Race and Wakeford, 2003; Rapp, 2000; Root and Browner, 2001). CATIE's own director of programme delivery, Darien Taylor, has been involved in research that points to the multiple and hybrid forms of knowledge that PLHIV engage in, the full conceptual and emotional repertoire with which they encounter it, their not uncommon indifference to text-based information and preference for face-to-face knowledge shared with those whom they know and trust (Making Care Visible Research Group, 2002). These insights have provoked a search within CATIE for new ways of thinking about the form and content of health information and its relationship to PLHIV, particularly those living in marginalised social and economic circumstances.

The development of CATIE as an organisation providing health information services to individual 'clients' also locates it in tension with neoliberal health reform. CATIE's organisational consolidation was coincident with the promotion on the part of health authorities in Canada and, indeed, across the global North of modes of self-governance predicated on the widespread distribution and consumption of health information. From the early 1990s, if not earlier, discourses of self-care, self-management and health information use proliferated as part of efforts to transform publicly funded health care into a private consumer good, cut funds from formal health care systems and promote individual responsibility for health (Armstrong et al., 2000; Crawford, 1994). CATIE's original vision was one of exchanging health information among various publics and communities, including within and across the health professions, community-based AIDS organisations and PLHIV. With success in procuring state funding, this vision evolved into one that was more focused on providing information to individual people living with HIV and AIDS conceptualised as consumers of information. CATIE thus faces an ongoing challenge of reinforcing its interest in intervening in the management of HIV and promoting a community-based politics of health empowerment, against different rationalities and techniques of health information marked by individualism, unrealistic obligations to personally manage health and the privileging of narrow models of rational, evidence-based decision making.

CATIE and integration

As someone who was involved with CATIE during the peak of activist critique of HIV prevention, I had anticipated that integration might be met by the organisation with considerable political controversy and debate. The language of integrating treatment and prevention has certainly entered CATIE. While there have been concerns raised that an emphasis on prevention may come at a loss or compromise of CATIE's historical focus on treatment information to PLHIV, the organisation's predominant response to integration thus far has been one of accommodation. CATIE has used integration as an organising concept to develop new directions in its programming that respond to tensions associated with its established orientation to treatment information and to extend its overall mission into areas that involve the provision of HIV prevention information.

While integration has not been a source of contention within CATIE, it carries implications for the kind of organisation CATIE will be and, more broadly, for the biopolitics of HIV and treatment, in particular how a community-based politics in pursuit of the health of people living with HIV and AIDS is imagined and practiced. CATIE's relationship to integration has been shaped by the complementary positioning of treatment and prevention that defines the space of integration discourse. However, important developments associated with integration, notably positive prevention and the use of ART as a prevention tool, unsettle that complementarity. They raise profound political questions about the role of PLHIV in preventing the transmission of HIV infection. They further point to emerging complexities involved in incorporating prevention into an organisational space that has defined treatment in relation to the health needs of HIV+ people.

Integration did not descend upon CATIE as a discrete and coherent discourse. It became organisationally present alongside other discursive influences in a gradual, somewhat muted fashion. One of the earliest moments of combining treatment and prevention information at CATIE occurred in two educational projects: Prefix, an information pamphlet for injection drug users and www.livepositive.ca, a website for youth. These two projects followed what one CATIE staff member described as encouragement for the organisation to broaden its concept of treatment to address 'everything that has to do with' living with HIV. Both projects included treatment information and information about testing for HIV and, in the case of Prefix, information on safe injection. Neither project was specifically conceptualised in relation to integration and while their novelty caught the attention of CATIE staff, their inclusion of prevention and treatment information was understood at the time as a matter of common sense. As one CATIE staff member put it, 'We couldn't give information about HIV treatment to young people without in some way talking about how HIV is transmitted .... It just didn't make a lot of sense.'

The beginnings of a more explicit appearance of integration discourse within CATIE arose as part of changes in funding. CATIE staff members recall thinking in earnest about the relationship between treatment and prevention as part of a 2003 application for renewed funding. Responding to this application was an important moment that pulled CATIE into the work of conceptualising itself in terms that would be accountable to a government policy goal of integration. Even at this stage, however, the organisational resonance of integration within CATIE was tenuous. As one staff member recalled, 'I remember that we did our entire submission and at the end, James made the remark, "I think the one thing we haven't done well is the integration of prevention and treatment"'.

Intrigued by the concept of integration and anticipating it might signal a new priority for state funders, Tiffany Veinot, CATIE's then director of information services, began researching the concept. Her research culminated in the publication of an article which is among the first attempts in the global North to articulate a community-based perspective on the integration of HIV treatment and prevention (Veinot, 2006). Veinot shared her developing thinking about integration and the final paper widely at CATIE, helping to establish the early parameters of thought about integration for the organisation. Veinot's analysis was largely framed within the predominant discourse of integration as a complementary relationship between treatment and prevention. In her paper, she argues that treatment and prevention should be considered points on a single continuum of illness prevention or prevention of negative health outcomes (Veinot, 2006). Veinot provides numerous examples of how prevention and treatment can be integrated and makes a strong call for integrating treatment, prevention and support in the delivery of community-based HIV services.

The most significant organisational presence of integration discourse within CATIE at the time of writing has occurred as part of the development and delivery of a project called 'Integrating HIV/AIDS Treatment Information, Prevention and Support Services Capacity Building Project'. The Project was launched in 2004 and is funded by the Public Health

Agency of Canada. The Capacity Building Project provides the clearest example of how CATIE has oriented to integration through organisational accommodation. Integration came to resonate for CATIE through the project not only for how it was drawn upon as a concept that helped to extend the reach of CATIE services, but also for how it helped resolve tensions in the organisation's established approach to providing HIV-related treatment information.

As the Capacity Building Project was being developed, CATIE had begun to consolidate its reputation as a national organisation. Located in Toronto – the largest city in Canada – CATIE faced the challenge of addressing HIV treatment information in a country with a vast territory where concerns had been expressed about the growing reach of HIV infection among women, new immigrants, youth, Aboriginals, injection drug users and other 'marginalized communities'. For example, while MSM have continued to represent the majority of HIV and AIDS diagnoses in Canada, currently accounting for 51% of prevalent cases of HIV (including AIDS) (Public Health Agency of Canada, 2007), by 2005 women accounted for some 20% of all HIV cases in Canada (including AIDS) (Public Health Agency of Canada, 2007) and Aboriginals, while making up just 3.3% of the total population, accounted for 7.5% of cases. At the same time, local epidemics continued in Toronto among MSM [13% prevalence rate (Myers et al., 2004)] and among IDU in Vancouver's inner city Downtown Eastside (18% prevalence rate) (Wood et al., 2008).

Multiple community-based AIDS organisations and initiatives, a number mirroring the sexual, gender, age and ethno-racial specificity of local epidemics had been established across the country's main urban centres. The majority of these organisations focused on prevention and support and lacked expertise and resources in HIV treatment information. At the same time, concerns had begun to be raised about the limitations of CATIE's established focus on biomedical information delivered through texts to individual users. While CATIE did a good job of reaching PLHIV who fashioned themselves as active users of health information, in order to reach those for whom HIV treatment information was a more distant reality, particularly HIV+ people from 'marginalized communities', new approaches would be required.

The Capacity Building Project responds to these tensions by conjoining the logic and techniques of capacity building with the discourse of integration. Rather than CATIE attempting to develop ways of providing treatment information to new communities of PLHIV on its own, the Project creates opportunities to work with local organisations, more knowledgeable about the life circumstances of their clients, to help them develop strategies of treatment information that are tailored to those circumstances and to local organisational exigencies. The Project is based on a series of workshops designed in collaboration with local organisations and delivered by CATIE staff to local participants over a two-day period. The workshop curriculum typically includes treatment information as well as exercises for exploring how treatment information can be better integrated with the existing prevention and support services of local organisations. In the Project's first phase, seven organisations across the country participated. All were located outside of major urban centres and worked with women, Aboriginals, gay men, the economically disadvantaged and other people living with HIV and AIDS. One of the most significant outcomes of the project has been the development of a distinct, community-based perspective on integration. That perspective orients to the question of how to better link community-based prevention and treatment-related activities to address client needs, rather than committing to integration as a principle of administrative efficiency, as is common in managerial discourse and practice (Mykhalovskiy et al., 2009).

The Capacity Building Project was an important initiative for CATIE that concretised the possibility of working with treatment information in a mode that focuses on enhancing organisational capacities rather than providing information to individual health consumers. The Project targets small frontline organizations and tries to enhance their capacities to better provide treatment information in ways that are adapted to local needs and circumstances rather than rely on standardised text information produced at a distance. Thus far, however, CATIE's own role in the Project has not strayed far from its established expertise of providing treatment information.

The muted presence of direct work on prevention at CATIE changed in 2007 when the organisation received funding from the Public Health Agency of Canada to expand its mandate to include the distribution of HIV prevention information. CATIE now represents itself a 'knowledge exchange broker' for HIV/AIDS information in Canada, offering 'information, resources and contacts addressing all aspects of HIV including treatment, prevention, care and support' (CATIE, 2008). This new role builds on CATIE's experience with the Capacity Building Project but positions the organisation to support frontline organisations in responding to HIV through enhanced treatment and prevention efforts. In the short time since CATIE has expanded its mandate it has trained staff to respond to prevention requests on its 1-800 enquiry service, amalgamated the prevention and other resources of the Canadian HIV/AIDS Information Centre within its own holdings, initiated a national survey of community-based organisations focused on their HIV prevention services and included new resources on its webpage dealing with HIV prevention.

CATIE, integration and the biopolitics of HIV

What is the significance of this shift for CATIE? How does it affect CATIE's organisational identity and the scope of its action and work? What implications does it hold for the organisation's historical relationship to a politics that links the object of health with biomedical treatments and an HIV-related disease and identity-based social movement?

At a basic level, CATIE's embrace of integration represents an undeniable break from its foundational politics. CATIE can no longer represent itself as an organisation that works for the improved health of PLHIV through a singular focus on treatment information. Assuming that a full refashioning of the organisation's identity is unlikely and undesirable, how CATIE will represent itself both with respect to the health of HIV+ people and to treatments as ongoing objects of political significance will be a challenge.

One option might be to reframe the political antagonism between treatment and prevention that was the organisation's founding impetus. Arguments might be made, for example, that in a context where relatively effective treatments are widely available, the health interests of HIV+ and HIV– people are no longer as distinct as they were at the outset of the epidemic. Prevention might be recast as fully compatible with the health concerns of PLHIV drawing on arguments, for example, that when HIV+ people engage in safer sex they protect themselves from potential co-infections (Wolitski et al. 2005). Extending the trope of complementarity, CATIE might represent its embrace of integration as a new 'win–win' situation for all.

Two important developments associated with integration – positive prevention and biomedical prevention, particularly the use of ART to prevent the sexual transmission of HIV – complicate the possibility of extending the complementarity of prevention and treatment in this way. Both developments raise tensions in the relationship between treatment and prevention at the locus of responsibility for HIV infection, calling attention to enduring complexities in the relationship between public health rationalities associated with prevention and a PLHIV-centred health activism broadly conceived. At the same time, both developments suggest new possibilities of response for CATIE that move the biopolitics of HIV and treatment in a new direction. That direction extends treatment politics from questions of access to questions that concern how treatments are implicated in new forms of responsibility for HIV transmission that centre on the conduct and bodies of HIV+ people.

Positive prevention is a term used to refer to a variety of initiatives that focus attention on people living with HIV and AIDS as participants or targets of HIV prevention (Kalichman, 2005). Positive prevention is an important development in the techniques and rationality of HIV prevention for how it reorients the enterprise from an established focus on HIV– people or 'the general public' to those already infected with HIV. An important impetus behind positive prevention has been governmental anxiety about the effects of ART. From the perspective of infectious disease control reasoning, ART extends the lives of PLHIV, creating a larger pool of HIV+ people with the capacity to transmit HIV. The central intent of early forms of positive prevention was to enlist PLHIV in efforts to stop the transmission of HIV.[5] Early proposals advancing positive prevention were made in the policy literature on integration. In an important statement, the Global HIV Prevention Working Group (2004: 14) noted that ART would likely help PLHIV 'recover sexual desire' and argued for prevention programmes directed at PLHIV that, among other measures, introduced new expectations for them to disclose their HIV status.

Biomedical prevention dates back to the use of AZT to prevent mother-to-child transmission of HIV (Sperling et al., 1996). More recently, researchers have argued that newer combinations of ART are so successful at reducing the amount of virus in the blood that they have a protective value against the sexual transmission of HIV (Quinn et al., 2000). In a recent statement, researchers from Switzerland's Federal AIDS Commission have gone so far as to state that under optimal conditions, HIV+ people with undetectable viral load cannot transmit the virus (Vernazza, Hirschel, Bernasconi and Flepp, 2008). Others such as Montaner and colleagues (Anema, Wood and Montaner, 2008; Montaner, 2006; Montaner et al., 2006) have put forward population-based models of ART-led prevention that argue for mass distribution and use of ART in developing countries to help prevent HIV transmission. These developments signal a profound shift in the established techniques of HIV prevention marked most importantly by an ontological shift in the status of ART. Formerly understood and enacted as a clinical treatment for HIV infection, ART is now routinely positioned discursively, if not yet fully in practice, as a prevention tool. As one might expect, a host of debates have followed focusing on such issues as the relative importance of biomedical and behavioural HIV prevention strategies (Kippax and Race, 2003; Paxton, Hope and Jaffe, 2007), the relationship between research on viral load and ART and increased uptake of 'high-risk behaviours'

(Crepaz, Hart and Marks, 2004; Stolte et al., 2004) and the tendency for biomedical prevention to support individualising, 'quick fix' approaches to the problem of HIV transmission (Imrie et al., 2007).

CATIE's primary response to these developments aligns with the established programmatic and political lineaments of its work on HIV treatment information. Thus, of the two developments, positive prevention and biomedical prevention, the latter has captured more attention from the organisation. In addressing the issues presented by positioning ART as a form of HIV prevention, CATIE has gravitated toward a familiar terrain – commentary and critique of scientific research on biomedical treatments, albeit with a focus on prevention. Thus CATIE's editor of *TreatmentUpdate*, Sean Hosein, has written an important article critiquing the scientific research upon which the Swiss Federal AIDS Commission study was based (Hosein, 2008). At the annual meetings of the Canadian Association for HIV/AIDS Research, CATIE organised a Learning Institute targeting a 'lay' audience of PLHIV and focused topically on biomedical prevention. Most of the speakers at the Learning Institute were physicians and clinical researchers who offered interpretations of the latest research on the preventive value of ART. The Learning Institute generated debate and discussion about whether ART should be understood as and used for HIV prevention. However, the discursive terrain of that debate was limited primarily to matters of scientific research.[6]

The shifting boundaries between treatment and prevention challenge CATIE's organisational repertoire. At a public level, like other nongovernmental organisations CATIE has responded to the possibility of treatments being used for prevention with caution, emphasising that treatments can never fully protect against HIV transmission and arguing for the need to maintain safe behaviours by following established behavioural prevention strategies. At the same time, CATIE staff recognise that in many contexts behavioural prevention has had limited success, that ART does have a measure of protection against HIV transmission and that a public discourse to that effect has begun to take hold. In a recent interview, one CATIE staff member noted with concern that some PLHIV now orient to ART not simply as a clinical resource but as something they should take in order to be 'less infectious'. This new enactment of biomedical treatment, one that emphasises preserving the HIV– status of others, suggests just how far we have come from the days when CATIE and other organisations formulated an activism around HIV treatments that aimed to intervene in the organisation of clinical care in the name of securing the health of PLHIV.

As important as CATIE's early responses to biomedical prevention have been, they do not fully address the historic repositioning of ART that is taking place within current developments associated with integration. Nor do they fully address the issues of concern presented to PLHIV in what some CATIE staff describe as a 'new era of treatments'. The questions provoked by positive prevention and biomedical prevention call for responses that exceed a community-based politics of critiquing and translating scientific discourse for lay audiences. They raise profound ethico-political questions about responsibility for HIV infection. One way CATIE can orient to integration while extending its historical emphasis on addressing the health issues faced by PLHIV is to more fully enter into debates about responsibility for HIV transmission that have been provoked by the integration of treatment and prevention.

Responsibility for HIV transmission has long been a site of contestation and transformation (Adam, 2006; Bloor, 1995; Dowsett, 1996; Kippax and Race, 2003; Patton, 1990; Scott and Freeman, 1995). Positive prevention and biomedical prevention contribute to these shifting relations by reconfiguring responsibility in ways that are centred on the figure of the person living with HIV, albeit in contradictory ways. Positive prevention is, in part, a project of governing HIV+ people in ways that align their conduct with a formative biopolitical identity. That identity departs considerably from that of the Foucauldian biological citizen who makes claims on health resources in the name of enhancing his or her health (Petryna, 2002; Rose, 2007). Positive prevention, by contrast, supports a subject for whom acting responsibly in matters of health is coordinated conceptually by concerns for the health of the population, manifested in securing the health of others by minimising the risk of HIV transmission to them.

These 'responsibilizing' effects of positive prevention suggest ongoing tensions in the relationship of treatment and prevention. A number of PLHIV groups have voiced concerns about how positive prevention initiatives organised by a 'public health control' perspective ignore the health needs of HIV+ people and take interest in them only as potential vectors of infection (Moody, 2007). A further tension emerging from positive prevention concerns how centring responsibility for HIV transmission on the conduct of PLHIV can erode earlier traditions emphasising mutual responsibility for HIV transmission on the part of both HIV+ and HIV– people. Making PLHIV primarily responsible for HIV transmission also creates new opportunities for stigmatising and discriminating against them.

Biomedical prevention also places new demands on PLHIV that are centred around the prevention of transmission. Research that suggests PLHIV with undetectable viral loads are unlikely to transmit HIV seemingly releases HIV+ people from responsibility for preventing HIV transmission. One of the remarkable features of attending the 2008 International AIDS Conference was witnessing the potential emergence of a new sexual subjectivity for PLHIV associated with the effects of ART on HIV transmission. At a session on the Swiss Federal AIDS Commission study, PLHIV in the audience rose to speak about their excitement about being able to have sex without constant worry about infecting their partners. It was a profound moment suggesting how biomedical research may contribute to breaking decades of association between sexual expression and the burden of HIV transmission for PLHIV.

At the same time, however, biomedical prevention has the potential to reinforce the centring of responsibility for HIV transmission in the individual bodies and conduct of PLHIV. Biomedical prevention can individualise HIV transmission, directing attention away from broad, social determinants of risk activities and the interpersonal and relational dynamics associated with HIV transmission. The positioning of ART as a prevention tool is part of a broader discourse of integration that problematises early 'HIV transmitters' – PLHIV who do not know their HIV status and engage in unsafe behaviours – and targets them for intervention through mandatory HIV testing, disclosure of HIV status, early commencement of biomedical therapy and ongoing behavioural risk reduction (Brenner et al., 2007; Wainberg, 2007). It thus coordinates social relations of engagement with biomedical treatment that intend a project of reducing HIV transmission centred on managing the behaviour of HIV+ people. Biomedical prevention potentially decouples treatment onset from clinical reasoning, encouraging PLHIV to begin taking ART because it will make them less infectious, rather than because it is clinically indicated. It also potentially introduces non-clinical considerations into treatment adherence. The consequences of these moves, particularly given the potential long-term side effects of ART, are cause for concern.

Positive prevention and biomedical prevention suggest important tensions in the relationship of HIV prevention and treatment at the site of PLHIV bodies and conduct that are given short shrift by a discourse of complementarity that characterises contemporary thought about integration. Drawing on my experiences with CATIE, I have argued that, in the Canadian context, integration disrupts the trope of complementarity in HIV integration discourse. The increasing association of treatment with prevention heightens HIV+ people's responsibility for the transmission of HIV infection, potentially exposing them to stigmatisation and discrimination, eroding public conceptions of shared responsibility for HIV transmission and destabilising treatment commencement and use from its base in clinical reasoning. The implications for how PLHIV are publicly understood and responded to by state and governmental health authorities in matters of HIV prevention loom large.

The stakes have only risen of late, with a growing global trend toward the criminalisation of HIV transmission (Burris and Cameron, 2008; UNAIDS, 2008). In parts of Africa, Asia, Latin America and the Caribbean, new HIV-specific laws have been introduced, while in Europe and North America existing legislation, often laws related to sexual assault and serious bodily harm, have been used to charge PLHIV for transmitting or exposing others to HIV (Open Society Institute, 2008). While the relevant legislation varies from country to country, it generally permits charges to be laid against HIV+ people for either 'knowingly' or 'willfully' transmitting HIV to a sexual partner or for failing to disclose their HIV status to sexual partners, regardless of whether HIV transmission has occurred. In some jurisdictions, the criminal law permits people to be charged whether or not they have been diagnosed HIV+. In Canada, PLHIV have a legal obligation to disclose their HIV+ status to people before engaging in activities that pose a 'significant risk' of transmitting HIV during sex (Canadian HIV Legal Network, 2008). At the time of writing, a flurry of charges in Canada in recent months has led to widespread concern among Canadian AIDS activists about the expansive use of criminal law in situations of HIV nondisclosure and its stigmatisation of PLHIV and impact on established public health approaches.[7]

The contradictory developments associated with thought and practice that link HIV treatment with prevention signal an important change in the biopolitics of AIDS. That change is characterised by a shift in the significance of treatments as a political object. The stabilisation of relatively successful biomedical therapy for HIV infection has calmed HIV treatment activism and movement organising in Canada. While hardly a final solution to the health challenges of HIV infection, the arrival of ART has displaced the 'golden bad old days' of a national HIV treatment activism in Canada. The political centre of treatment activism has shifted to issues of globalisation and access to ART in developing countries. While the old days of HIV treatment activism may have passed, CATIE and organizations like it need not fully abandon political commitments to acting in what might be considered the health interests of PLHIV, however diverse the latter may be. Still, CATIE's embrace of integration requires responses that transcend a focus on HIV treatment information animated by a politics of empowerment and realised programmatically through the democratisation of scientific knowledge. Integration invites CATIE to intervene in public debate about the reconfiguration of responsibility for HIV transmission, particularly in ways that are mindful of the potential effects on PLHIV. Given the rather dramatic shifts that have occurred and the complex ways in which clinical and public health reasoning and techniques are interacting as treatments are being aligned with the goals of preventing HIV transmission there will be a need for a strong community voice to help PLHIV and others navigate the waters.

Conclusion

This chapter has argued that the established discourse on integration offers a narrow conceptualisation of the articulation of biomedicine and public health at the site HIV, positioning treatment and prevention as co-supportive with near unbridled enthusiasm and a marked absence of reflexivity. Drawing on the work of Flyvbjerg, I have opened up a space for considering the broader variety of ways that HIV treatment and prevention may be related with one another, including forms of association that involve relations of tension and conflict. The point has not been to argue for tension over complementarity, but to provide a context-specific analysis of one response to integration and its potential effects on community-based treatment service and politics. Policy-making geared into the notion of an inevitable complementary relationship between treatment and prevention and supported by overly general levels of analysis, comparative or otherwise, need to be replaced by thinking that explores how connections between local epidemics, state and professional responses to HIV, the availability of treatment and prevention, the history of AIDS activism and other factors shape how integration is enacted and with what effect.

References

Adam, B. (2006) 'Infectious behaviour: imputing subjectivity to HIV transmission', *Social Theory and Health*, 4, 168–79.

Anema, A., Wood, E. and Montaner, J. (2008) 'The use of highly active retroviral therapy to reduce HIV incidence at the population level', *Canadian Medical Association Journal*, 179, 1, 13–14.

Armstrong, P., Armstrong, H., Bourgeault, I., Choiniere, J., Mykhalovskiy, E. and White, M. (2000) *Heal thyself: managing health care reform* (Toronto: Garamond Press).

Biehl, J. (2008) 'Drugs for all: the future of global AIDS treatment', *Medical Anthropology*, 27, 2, 99–105.

Binder, L. (2006) 'From programmes to policies now: positive changes for women and girls', International AIDS Conference, Plenary session, August 14.

Bloor, M (1995) 'A user's guide to contrasting theories of HIV-related risk behaviour', in J. Gabe (ed.) *Medicine, health and risk: sociological approaches* (Oxford: Blackwell).

Brenner, B., Roger, M., Routy, J., Moisi, D., Ntemgwa, M. Matte, C., Baril, J. G., Thomas, R., Rouleau, D., Bruneau, J., Leblanc, R., Legault, M., Tremblay, C., Charest, H. and Wainberg, M. A. (2007) 'High rates of forward transmission events after acute/early HIV-1 infection', *The Journal of Infectious Diseases*, 195, 951–9.

Burris, S. and Cameron, E. (2008) 'The case against criminalization of HIV transmission', *Journal of the American Medical Association*, 300, 5, 578–80.

Cain, R. (2002) 'Devoting ourselves, devouring each other: tensions in community-based AIDS work', *Journal of Progressive Human Services*, 13, 1, 93–113.

Canadian HIV/AIDS Legal Network (2008) 'Criminal law and HIV', http://www.aidslaw.ca/publications/interfaces/downloadFile.php?ref=1318, July 10, 2008.

CATIE (2008) 'Our changing role', http://www.catie.ca/eng/AboutCATIE/ChangingRole.shtml, July 1, 2008.

Crawford, R. (1994) 'The boundaries of the self and the unhealthy other: reflections on health, culture, and AIDS', *Social Science & Medicine*, 38, 1347–65.

Crepaz, N., Hart, T. and Marks, G. (2004) 'Highly active antiretroviral therapy and sexual risk behaviour: a meta-analytic review', *Journal of the American Medical Association*, 292, 2, 224–36.

De Cock, K. (2006) 'From "3 by 5" to universal access', International AIDS Conference, Plenary session, August 16.

Dowsett, G. (1996) *Practicing desire: homosexual sex in the era of AIDS* (Stanford: Stanford University Press).

Epstein, S. (1996) *Impure science: AIDS activism and the politics of knowledge* (Berkeley: University of California Press).

—— (2000) 'Democracy, expertise and AIDS treatment activism', in D. Kleinman (ed.) *Science, Technology and Democracy* (Albany: Suny Press).

Farmer, P. (2006 [1992]) *AIDS and accusation: Haiti and the geography of blame* (Berkeley: University of California Press).

—— (2003) 'AIDS as a global emergency', *Bulletin of the World Health Organization*, 81, 10, 699.

Farmer, P., Leandre, F., Mukherjee, J., Claude, M., Nevil, P., Smith-Fawzi, M., Koenig, S., Castro, A., Becerra, M., Sachs, J., Attaran, A. and Kim, J. (2001) 'Community-based approaches to HIV treatment in resource-poor settings', *The Lancet*, 358, 404–9. Ferzacca, S. (2000) '"Actually, I don't feel that bad": managing diabetes and the clinical encounter', *Medical Anthropology Quarterly*, 14, 1, 28–50.

Flyvbjerg, B. (2001) *Making social science matter: why social inquiry fails and how it can succeed again* (Cambridge: Cambridge University Press).

Gayle, H. and Lange, J. (2004) 'Seizing the opportunity to capitalise on the growing access to HIV treatment to expand HIV prevention', *The Lancet*, 364, 9428, 6–8.

Global HIV Prevention Working Group (2004) *HIV prevention in the era of expanded treatment access*, www.gatesfoundation.org, August 1, 2008.

Hassan, F. (2006) 'Getting the balance right: integrating HIV prevention and treatment programming: a panel discussion', International AIDS Conference, August 14.

Health Canada (n.d.) 'Canada's health care system (medicare)', http://www.hc-sc.gc.ca/hcs-sss/medi-assur/index-eng.php, January 15, 2009.

Hosein, S. (2008) 'Swiss guidelines take a troubling turn', http://www.catie.ca/eng/WhatsNew/WhatsNewIndex.shtml, June 28, 2008.

Imrie, J., Elford, J., Kippax, S. and Hart, G. (2007) 'Biomedical prevention – and social science', *The Lancet*, 370, 10–11.

International HIV/AIDS Alliance (2003) 'Positive prevention: prevention strategies for people with HIV/AIDS, draft background paper', http://www.aidsalliance.org/graphics/secretariat/publications/ppr0703_positive_prevention.pdf, June 9, 2008.

Kalichman, S. (ed.) (2005) *Positive prevention: reducing HIV transmission among people living with HIV/AIDS* (New York: Kluwer Academic/Plenum Publishers).

Kippax, S. and Race, S. (2003) 'Sustaining safe practice: twenty years on', *Social Science & Medicine*, 57, 1–12.

Koenig, S., Leandre, F. and Farmer, P. (2004) 'Scaling-up HIV treatment programmes in resource-limited settings: the rural Haiti experience', *AIDS*, 18, Suppl. 3, S21–S25.

Kort, R., Flynn, M., Gilden, D., Mascolini, M., Mykhalovskiy, E., Baijal, P. and Brown, G. (2008) *The AIDS 2008 impact report: evidence to action* (Geneva: International AIDS Society), http://www.iasociety.org/Web/WebContent/File/AIDS%202008_impact_report.pdf .

Making Care Visible Research Group (Bresalier, M., Gillis, L., McClure, C., McCoy, L., Mykhalovskiy, E., Taylor, D. and Webber, M.) (2002) *Making care visible: antiretroviral therapy and the health work of people living with HIV/AIDS*. A research report funded by the Positive Action Fund, administered by the AIDS Program Committee, AIDS Bureau, Ontario Ministry of Health.

McCoy, L. (2005) 'HIV positive patients and the doctor–patient relationship: perspectives from the margins', *Qualitative Health Research*, 15, 6, 791–806.

Montaner, J., Hogg, R., Wood, E., Kerr, E., Tyndall, M., Levy, A. (2006) 'The case for expanding access to highly active antiretroviral therapy to curb the growth of the HIV epidemic', *The Lancet*, 368, 9534, 531–6.

Montaner, J. (2006) 'Re-evaluating the cost-effectiveness of HAART: the case for expanding treatment access to curb the growth of the epidemic', International AIDS Conference, Plenary Session, August 16.

Moody, K. (2007) 'Positive prevention: opportunity or threat', http://www.healthdev.org/eforums/cms/individual.asp?sid=183&sname=Accelerating-Prevention, November 5, 2008.

Mukherjee, J. and Eustache, F. (2007) 'Community health workers as a cornerstone for integrating HIV and primary healthcare', *AIDS Care*, 19, Suppl. 1, S73–82.

Myers, T., Allman, D., Calzavarra, L., Maxwell, J., Remis, R., Swantee, C. and Travers, R. (2004). *The Ontario men's survey* (Toronto: HIV Social, Behavioural, and Epidemiological Studies Unit, University of Toronto), http://www.mens-survey.ca/doc/OMS_Report_web_final%20.pdf, January 10, 2009.

Mykhalovskiy, M., McCoy, L. and Bresalier, M. (2004) 'Compliance/adherence, HIV/AIDS and the critique of medical power', *Social Theory and Health*, 2, 4, 315–40.

Mykhalovskiy, M. (2008) 'Beyond decision making: class, community organizations and the healthwork of people living with HIV/AIDS: contributions from institutional ethnographic research', *Medical Anthropology: Cross Cultural Studies in Health and Illness*, 27, 2, 136–63.

Mykhalovskiy, E., Patten, S., Sanders, C., Bailey, M. and Taylor, D. (2009) 'Conceptualizing the integration of HIV treatment and prevention: findings from a process evaluation of a community-based, national capacity-building intervention', *International Journal of Public Health* 54, 3, 133–41.

Mykhalovskiy, M., Patten, S., Sanders, C., Bailey, M. and Taylor, S. (2009) 'Beyond buzzwords: towards a community-based model of the integration of HIV treatment and prevention', *AIDS Care*, 21, 1, 25–30.

Ontario Ministry of Health and Long-term Care (n.d.) 'Ontario drug benefit: Trillium drug program', http://www.health.gov.on.ca/english/public/pub/drugs/trillium.html, January 19, 2009.

Open Society Institute (2008) '10 reasons why criminalization of HIV exposure or transmission is bad public policy', www.aidsportal.org/repos/10reasonsdraft_20080918.pdf, January 10, 2009.

Patton, C. (1990) *Inventing AIDS* (New York/London: Routledge).

Paxton, L., Hope, T. and Jaffe, H. (2007) 'Pre-exposure prophylaxis for HIV infection: what if it works?', *The Lancet*, 370, 9581, 89–93.

Persson, A., Race, K. and Wakeford, E. (2003) 'HIV health in context: negotiating medical technology and lived experience', *Health: An Interdisciplinary Journal for the Social Study of Health, Illness and Medicine*, 7, 4, 397–415.

Petryna, A. (2002) *Life exposed: biological citizens after Chernobyl* (Princeton: Princeton University Press).

Public Health Agency of Canada (2007) *HIV epi updates*, November (Ottawa: Surveillance and Risk Assessment Division, Centre for Infectious Disease Prevention and Control).

Quinn, T., Wawer, M., Sewankambo, N., Serwadda, D., Li, C., Wabwire-Mangen, F., Meehan, M., Lutalo, T. and Gray, R. (2000) 'Viral load and heterosexual transmission of human immunodeficiency virus type 1, Rakai project study group', *New England Journal of Medicine*, 30, 342, 13, 921–9.

Rapp, R. (2000) 'Extra chromosomes and blue tulips: medico-familial interpretations', in M. Lock, A. Cambrosio and A. Young (eds) *Living and working with the new medical technologies: intersections of inquiry* (New York: Cambridge University Press).

Root, R. and Browner, C. (2001) 'Practices of the pregnant self: compliance with and resistance to prenatal norms', *Culture, Medicine and Psychiatry*, 25, 2, 195–223.

Rose, N. (2007) *The politics of life itself. Biomedicine, power, and subjectivity in the twenty-first century* (Princeton: Princeton University Press).

Salomon, S., Hogan, D., Stover, J., Stanecki, K., Walker, N., Ghys, P. and Schwartländer, B. (2005) 'Integrating HIV prevention and treatment: from slogans to impact', *PLoS Medicine*, 2, 1, e16, 50–6.

Schwartländer, B., Grubb, I. and Perriëns, J. (2006) 'The 10-year struggle to provide antiretroviral treatment to people with HIV in the developing world', *Lancet*, 368, 541–6.

Scott, S. and Freeman, R. (1995) 'Prevention as a problem of modernity: the example of HIV and AIDS', in J. Gabe (ed.) *Medicine, Health and Risk: Sociological Approaches* (Oxford: Blackwell).

Shodell, D. (2006) 'Global treatment for HIV/AIDS: integrating prevention in the wake of "3 by 5"', *Medscaple Public Health & Prevention*, http://www.medscape.com/viewarticle/530941?rss, June 11, 2008.

Simao, M. (2006) 'Getting the balance right: integrating HIV prevention and treatment programming: a panel discussion', International AIDS Conference, August 14.

Smith, G. (1990) 'Political activist as ethnographer', *Social Problems*, 37, 4, 629–48.

—— (2005) 'Accessing treatments: managing the AIDS epidemic in Ontario', in M. Campbell and A. Manicom (eds) *Knowledge, experience and ruling relations: studies in the social organization of knowledge* (Toronto: University of Toronto Press).

Smith, R. and Siplon, P. (2006). *Drugs into bodies: global AIDS treatment activism* (Westport: Praeger).

Sperling, R., Shapiro, D., Coombs, R., Todd, J., Herman, S., McSherry, G., O'Sullivan, M., Van Dyke, R., Jimenez, E., Rouzioux, C., Flynn, P. and Sullivan, J. (1996) 'Maternal viral load, zidovudine treatment, and the risk of transmission of human immunodeficiency virus type 1 from mother to infant', *New England Journal of Medicine*, 335, 22, 1621–9.

Statistics Canada (2009) 'Canada's population estimates', http://www.statcan.gc.ca/daily-quotidien/081219/dq081219b-eng.htm, January 19, 2009.

Stolte, I., Dukers, N., Geskus, R., Coutinho, R. and de Wit, J. (2004) 'Homosexual men change to risky sex when perceiving less threat of HIV/AIDS since availability of highly active antiretroviral therapy: a longitudinal study', *AIDS*, 18, 2, 303–9.

UNAIDS (2008) 'Criminalization of HIV transmission policy brief', http://data.unaids.org/pub/BaseDocument/2008/20080731_jc1513_policy_criminalization_en.pdf, January 10, 2009.

Veinot, T. (2006) 'The case for an integrated approach to HIV/AIDS prevention, support and treatment services in Canada', *Journal of HIV/AIDS & Social Services*, 5, 3/4, 181–99.

Vernazza, P., Bernasconi, E., Hirschel, B. and Flepp, M. (2008) 'Les personnes séropositives ne souffrant d'aucune autre MST et suivant un traitement antirétroviral efficace ne transmettent pas le VIH par voie sexuelle', *Bulletin des Médecins Suisses*, 89, 5, 165–9.

Wainberg, W. (2007) 'New HIV transmission in Canada: concerns regarding drug resistance and the failure of prevention', keynote address, *RBC conference forty million and counting: cutting edge challenges in HIV prevention*, University of Toronto, Canada, November 15.

Walton, D., Farmer, P., Lambert, W., Leandre, F., Koenig, S. and Mukherjee, J. (2004) 'Integrated HIV prevention and care strengthens primary health care: lessons from rural Haiti', *Journal of Public Health Policy*, 25, 2, 137–58.

Wood, E., Montaner, J., Li, K., Zhang, R., Barney, L., Strathdee, S., Tyndall, M. and Kerr, T. (2008) 'Burden of HIV infection among aboriginal injection drug users in Vancouver, British Columbia', *American Journal of Public Health*, 98, 3, 515–19.

WHO and UNAIDS (2006) 'Progress on global access to HIV antiretroviral therapy: a report on "3 by 5" and beyond', www.who.int/hiv/fullreport_en_highres.pdf.

Wolitski, R., Janssen, R., Onorato, I., Purcell, D. and Crepaz, N. (2005) 'An overview of prevention with people living with HIV', in S. Kalichman (ed.) *Positive prevention: reducing HIV transmission among people living with HIV/AIDS* (New York: Kluwer Academic/Plenum Publishers).

Notes

I would like to thank the editors, Corinne Squire and Mark Davis, for their helpful comments on an earlier version of this chapter. Darien Taylor and Tim Rogers offered useful critiques and suggestions as I formulated the chapter's argument.

I would also like to thank the people whose interviews are drawn upon in this chapter. All proper names are changed in quoted material. The writing of this article was supported by a Social Science and Humanities Research Council Standard Research Grant (410-2005–2003) and a New Investigator Award from the Canadian Institutes of Health Research.

1. The 3 by 5 initiative was established by WHO and UNAIDS in 2003. Its objective was to provide three million people living with HIV and AIDS access to ART by 2005. For details see WHO and UNAIDS (2006).
2. Interestingly, the conceptualization of integration as a complementary relationship between HIV prevention and HIV treatment, was extended at the 2008 International AIDS Conference held in Mexico to address challenges posed about the broader health services and development impact of global HIV-specific funding initiatives. A number of sessions were held at the conference to debate and counter claims that HIV-specific development assistance is poorly integrated with general health systems strengthening. One of the central mantras at the 2008 conference was the need to continue to develop approaches that integrate HIV-specific initiatives with primary health care and general health care system reform and development. See Kort et al. (2008).
3. In Canada, the delivery, organization and management of health services are a provincial responsibility. The principles of Canada's publicly insured health care system are outlined in the Canada Health Act (1985). Canada's "national system" is, in practice, a system of interlinked provincial and territorial insurance plans that provide medically necessary physician and hospital care financed through taxation rather than point of care contributions from patients. Pharmaceutical treatments administered outside of Canadian hospital settings are funded for those in need through a variety of provincial plans with different levels of coverage, eligibility requirements, premiums and deductibles (Health Canada, n.d.). In Ontario, PLHIV who have "high prescription drug costs in relation to their net household income can access HIV-related medications through the Trillium Drug Program" (Ontario Ministry of Health and Long-term Care, n.d.).
4 Tim McCaskell, personal communication, 10 June 2008.
5. Positive prevention is contested terrain. In response to narrow early formulations that privilege the question of transmission, PLHIV groups and community-based AIDS organizations have argued for a broader notion of positive prevention that includes a vision of "healthy living" for PLHIV, freedom from stigmatization and discrimination, access to needed services and a broad understanding of the social context of HIV risk. See, for example, International HIV/AIDS Alliance, 2003.
6. The debate centred on two central issues: (1) how to interpret population-level studies in contexts of individual risk behaviour, (2) the potential importance for transmission of HIV in seminal fluid vs. blood.
7. The Ontario Working Group on Criminal Law and HIV Exposure was established in Toronto in 2007 to spearhead a provincial campaign to oppose the expansive application of criminal law in situations of HIV nondisclosure.

5

Parental Communication with Children about Sex in the HIV/AIDS Epidemic in South Africa: Cultural Appropriations of Western Parenting Expertise

Lindy Wilbraham

Western parenting expertise in African HIV/AIDS epidemic

The South African HIV/AIDS epidemic has heterosexually active people at its demographic epicentre; and within the power relations of gender, resource-poverty and hetero-normative sexual culture, women of child-bearing age bear the brunt of sexual risk, HIV infection, illness, caring for those living with AIDS and death (Walker and Gilbert, 2002). Mothering has also come under surveillance in public health research due to the negative effects of the HIV epidemic on children's lives (see Foster, Levine and Williamson, 2005), and the apparently HIV-risk protective effects that are associated with certain childrearing practices. Talking about sex with children in particular ways, establishing warm relationships with them, and co-regulating and monitoring their activities are promised – in expert technological interventions to assist floundering parents – to scaffold responsible, risk-averse sexualities in young people *before* they are heterosexually active (e.g. Bhana et al., 2004; Blake et al., 2001; Grunseit et al., 1997). A Foucauldian perspective connects 'government' by the western *psy-complex* of the micro-practices of parenting with broader orders of public health, social stability and economic security (Burman, 2008; Lupton and Tulloch, 1998; Rose, 1990, 2007). This chapter explores how HIV prevention technologies require and fabricate particular kinds of sexual citizenship in parents and children.

In South Africa's conditions of post-apartheid transition and advanced HIV/AIDS epidemic, disparate access to resources still define communities. Idealised parenting technologies of the western *psy-complex* are largely assumed to hold in raced-white, middle-classed families, and to mono-causally explain lower HIV prevalence within these domestic cells. Thus risk-safety appears as an expression of the psychological techniques of mothering, rather than the economic benefits such neighbourhoods sustain (Rose, 2007). Against this idealised value, South African risk-prevention literatures recycle concerns about negative psychological impacts on classed-poor and raced-black children in adverse social conditions, with implications of inadequate custodial care, resources and socialisation provided by stretched, stricken or absent parents (Dawes and Donald, 1994). Inextricably woven into such poverty, traditional African cultural parenting practices are judged – by western *psy-complex* standards – as authoritarian and neglectful towards children and youth (Richter, 1994). Such risk-saturated parenting deficits attract globally funded research that aims to install healthier practices in order to manage risk, re-establish parental responsibilities and restore children's rights. This research is invariably fixated on dysfunctional communication about sex in resource-poor and raced-black families, with young people repeatedly figured as dissatisfied with parental preaching about reproduction, their scare tactics and their 'silence' about sex (e.g. Campbell, 2003; Kelly, Parker and Oyosi, 2001; *loveLife*, 2000a); and parents as ignorant, confused, ambivalent, reluctant or ineffectual communicators about sex with children (e.g. Paruk et al., 2005).

Such findings speak to the difficult place of *psy-complex* expertise in HIV literatures in this parenting field across the global/local epidemic in relation to resource poor and at-risk people (including those in the developed world). In South Africa, the implicit 'parent blaming' or 'culture-blaming' inherent in *psy-complex* expertise has had some arguably positive spin-offs in the generation of custodian-, youth- and community-targeted complex interventions involving various media and intersecting layers of participation, to fabricate the 'modern' communication skills required for authoritative management of young people's sexual socialisation (Bhana et al., 2004; Campbell, 2003; Kelly et al., 2001). These interventions explicitly engage, and seek to normalise, deleterious cultures, norms, relationships and choices in lived everyday contexts.

Although this chapter moves through similar territory, it engages with 'research on HIV/AIDS' in ways that critically interrogate what counts as knowledge, why, and how and on/with whom it is used. This chapter seeks to *localise* acculturated parenting practices around a *particular* HIV technology, in closer detail. Its discourse analytical readings unpack how a *particular* audience of well-educated, largely middle-classed, raced-black mothers appropriated psychological expertise on sex communication with children; and how they were directed towards subjective positions and practices in relation to risk-safety from HIV/AIDS, and their own lived experience as mothers and children. The chapter's discussants were given a short didactic text to talk about in groups. This text was a fragment of the broader *loveLife* campaign in South Africa, which, sometimes controversially, uses class-aspirational, sexual risk-prevention messaging to shape an 'HIV-free generation' of young brand-conscious consumers as heterosexual subjects/citizens (Thomas, 2004). *LoveLife* incorporates campaigning around the opening up of communication between parents and 'teenagers' (see *loveLife*, 2000a, 2000b); and this chapter is drawn from my wider attention to textual, discursive and socio-cultural practices pertaining to the *Lovelines* series on parenting responsibilities in an HIV/AIDS epidemic (see Wilbraham, 2002, 2004, 2008, 2009). This *loveLife*-collaborative series appeared in *Fairlady*, a nationally distributed, South African women's magazine which targeted mostly *middle-classed* mothers as its primary audience of reading subjects.

The *Lovelines* series, and my discussion groups about it, ran in 2000, which, of course, pre-dated establishment of broader antiretroviral treatment policies, roll-outs and services in South Africa. This historicity inevitably limited discursive resources available to campaigners and discussants alike, and heavily weighted HIV-prevention imperatives, seemingly severed from workable treatment options, in a *do-or-die* way. This do-or-die discourse is reproduced through the continuing unevenness of access to antiretroviral treatment in South Africa. My intention in this chapter is to explore – within the conditions of a heterosexually transmitted epidemic – how western, modern or expert parenting technologies were appropriated into local cultural practices in diverse South African communities and raced-black families. This attention focuses on the uneasily shifting power relations between 'African culture', 'race' and 'class-mobility' in mothering practices, and how sexual socialisation of children – or *the pedagogisation of sex* in Foucault's (1978) terminology – is/was done. As such, the chapter aligns itself theoretically and methodologically with critical discursive work on *subjectification* by reading the operation of expertise in media discourse to persuade and produce responsible sexual citizens, and so to govern risk. These 'lenses' are explicated below.

Media discourse as subjective and social government

Foucault's notion of *governmentality* unpicks how disciplinary powers of modern government work through the routine management of the minutiae of our lives, from a distance, through our reliance on 'facts' of scientific research and 'know-how' of expertise to avoid risk (Rose, 1992). Rose (1990) reads the *western psy-complex* – a historicised assemblage of institutions and technologies of the self with the *psy*-prefix: psychiatry, psychotherapy, psychoanalysis, child psychology – as fabricating a hegemonic currency of normal and preferred kinds of persons, conducts and relationships. This expertise is regulatory; but is beneficently geared towards facilitating individual development and healthful experience, and normalising troublesome problems of maladjustment and risk that threaten to destabilise populations (Rose, 1998). Such self-regulative beneficence is theorised as contingent on uncertain knowledge, resistance, constant vigilance and disciplinary work. However, the optimisation of subjective experience offered by expert technologies is crucial in understanding their powers to draw subjects, willingly, into government of their own and their children's conduct (Dean, 1994).

Feminist and discursive critiques have formulated the regulation of good mothering through psychological discourses about childrearing along these lines, pointing to how mothers are blamed when child development 'goes wrong' (see Alldred, 1996; Burman, 1994). Increasingly with the rise of modern institutional government, the *psy-complex* has powered legal, educational and social welfare agendas of child protection, and concerns about children's risk-safety, well-being and rights (Stainton-Rogers and Stainton-Rogers, 1992). Such shifts obviously pathologise, responsibilise and pedagogise mothering in powerful ways. A Foucauldian-feminist argument finds mothers positioned as relay points between 'public' (political, economic, social) and 'private' (family, emotions, sex) apparatuses; where their docile childrearing work according to contemporary *psy-complex* praxes is promised to produce healthy, autonomous, responsible young citizens (Walkerdine and Lucey, 1989). In extending this argument into an advanced HIV/AIDS epidemic in South Africa, this chapter considers how certain western parenting techniques – such as talking about sex with children – have become coupled to gender, class and risk-safety, and are seen as 'modern' and 'progressive' forms of biological citizenship (Rose, 2007).

Consideration of how 'persuasion' of maternal subjects works draws on particular strands of argument about *subjectification* through the operation of mass media discourse. Attention to media discourse seems to assume that media produces 'significant effects'; but, of course, there is little agreement on these effects (McQuail, 1994). In South African public health literatures on health-didactic media reception, there is disillusionment about the effectiveness of mass media campaigning – as a stand-alone HIV-prevention technology – to impart measurable skills, change behaviours or challenge norms in niche-specific ways that re-fabricate inclusive participatory dialogues and safer sexual activity (e.g. Bhana et al., 2004; Campbell, 2003; LeClerc-Madlala, 2002; Parker, 2003). Marxist and postmodern theoretical writings have polarised thinking about media reception into unhelpful binary positions, such as 'media power' which sticks duped subjects to certain ideological meanings/actions, or 'people power' where subjects are allowed untrammeled interpretive freedom and agency to appropriate what they want, resist or read against the grain (Hall, 1997).

In the instance of *purposive health-didactic texts*, such as those HIV-prevention technologies that seek to install 'proper-parenting', preferred meanings and techniques are wittingly encoded and distributed with particular audiences of subjects in mind (Fairclough, 1995; Miller et al., 1998; Mills, 1994). Fairclough (1992) argues that practices of media text consumption circle around the principle of '*coherence*': a coherent text is one whose representations of problems and advocated solutions are encoded to 'make sense' and 'persuade', even though there may be few formal markers of this coercive persuasion. Thus, Wilton (1997: 7) reads didactic texts on safer sex as deliberately encoded with the politics of gender, class, sexualities and risk-safety, and as 'instrumental to the constitution of subjectivities and social norms', because we mediate the kind of person we are and will/could be through the address and packaging of knowledge and actions made available to us.

The unease about didactic texts circles around the potential for slippages of persuasion and resistances to subjection by preferred practices (Blackman and Walkerdine, 2001); or in other words, that 'people power' to resist messaging overpowers 'media power' to predetermine meaning/action. With reference to this anxiety about slippage, this chapter attends to how the rhetorical and ideological surfaces of 'persuasion' (or subjectification) work partially, in piecemeal fashion; and are constantly re-negotiated in interactions with others through problematisation and advocacy of options, and performance, transmutation and appropriation of multivalent positions (Fairclough, 1992). Readers are subjected to/by expert technologies to the extent that preferred positions make sense within their own lived experience, and they are able to take up bits and pieces of advocated practices. Wetherell's (1998) discourse analytical approach, which is followed in this chapter, considers how gendered, raced, acculturated and/or classed speakers account for themselves in particular conversational contexts – for example, justify, defend, negotiate, contradict or resist particular positions based on their contextualised experience – against wider social and institutional discursive resources that regulate subjectivities, choices and agency.

Appropriating subjects and narratives about childrearing

This study asked groups of Southern African parents to read and discuss a *Lovelines* text, in relation to parenting practices they experienced with their own parents, and deploy with their own children. This produced opportunities for exploration both of the power of normative technologies of mothering and risk-safety, and their situated use, contestation and uncertainty. Fairclough (1992: 80) has drawn attention to the subtle interplay in practices of appropriation of didactic texts between (1) the *text* itself, as a particular set of problems, solutions and techniques; (2) the *reader's resources*, such as their cultural, educational, and media-literacy experiences, that are brought to text processing and (3) the *context of interpretation* that produces resources for normative, playful or oppositional readings. I will mention these praxes to account for how the particular group discussions were set up, before proceeding with an analysis of subject positioning.

Text

A single *Lovelines* text about talking with children about sex was selected to stimulate reflective discussion in groups – *Straight Talk* (*Fairlady*, 5 July 2000: 156). This 500-word text was not selected on the basis of it being typical of didactic discourse within *Fairlady* or *loveLife*, but as an HIV-prevention technology, it held together particular pedagogical (and rhetorical) issues I wished to explore in risk- and parenting expertise, most particularly the use of real life stories, statistical incidence rates of HIV/AIDS and teenage pregnancy as scare tactics, and actual topics and talking-techniques for communication with children. *Straight Talk* begins thus:

> Does your teenage daughter know when you had sex for the first time and with whom? Does she know whether you liked it? If the thought of discussing such intimate details with your child makes you cringe, consider that before she can turn to you for advice on sexual matters, she needs to know that you've had to make the same difficult choices and that you can relate to her.
>
> Every mother dreads the day when she must start talking to her teenagers about sex. But experts say if you wait until they're teenagers, you've waited too long. It should be an 18-year conversation

> about love, relationships, values and sex that begins as soon as your child starts to communicate. Before you begin to discuss sexual issues, be clear about your own values, but avoid coming across as pedantic and authoritarian.
>
> As a parent you must make an effort to understand and be willing to talk about the issues your daughter's grappling with, many of which may make you feel uncomfortable. These could include questions like: How do I know if I'm in love? Will sex bring me closer to my boyfriend? How do I know when I'm ready to have sex? Will having sex make me popular or will boys think I'm a slut? How do I tell my boyfriend I don't want to have sex without losing him? How does contraception work?

Attention to a single text focused discussion within and between groups, and selection of other mass media texts would produce different conversations. The participants were asked to read/discuss the text against their own experiences of childrearing and risk as children and as parents; and these transcribed narratives constituted 'texts' for analysis. This tactic is aligned with media reception studies that introduce specific materials to generate in-depth, interactive interpretations and struggle over meanings (Hermes, 1995). My epistemological intent in this chapter is avowedly not assessment of parents' knowledge, attitudes or behaviour – neither an attempt to change these; it is not a formal evaluation of the efficacy of *Lovelines*, *Fairlady* or *loveLife* in producing preferred meanings and parenting practices; and it is not a systematic media reception study.

Readers/discussants

Convenience sampling constituted heterogeneous discussion groups. The five groups involved participants who were senior postgraduate students and professional schoolteachers or university lecturers registered for a research methodology module on which I taught discourse analysis. Most participants were older than 35 years, were parents (only two were not) and were broadly middle-classed. Beyond these similarities, socio-cultural and discursive schisms appeared between genders; between mothers, fathers and 'childfree-subjects'; between postgraduate students, schoolteachers and academics; and between various African nationalities, cultural backgrounds and races. These heterogeneities were mixed across groups that ranged from two to six participants. This chapter does not seek to summarise the shifting themes and complex interactions of these discussions, but selects fragments of raced-black

South African mothers' stories in an analysis of appropriation of western parenting expertise against local/cultural practices. To uphold anonymity, pseudonyms are used in the extracts and some details of biographical or subjective reference were altered. The marking of racial and acculturated positioning of discussants was integral to a postcolonial argument about sex communication with children 'becoming white/r' within conditions of modernisation and class mobility in newly democratised South Africa (see Stoler, 1995).

Reading contexts

The context of reading *Straight Talk* was a practical workshop on discourse analysis in the above-mentioned postgraduate module on research methodology. The scaffolding of discussions within this intellectual context produced significant ruptures from 'ordinary talk' or 'natural discourse'. For example, individual mothers might read women's magazines at home, in waiting rooms or on buses, but my study 're-contextualized the discursive event' (Fairclough, 1995: 41) by placing consumption in an interpretive context of accountability to others, reflexivity and critique. Students and academics' familiarity with one another and the registers of 'academic debate' inscribed within a university context manufactured trust *and* defensiveness in revelation of their own experiences and adversarial positioning. It is unclear whether discussants were already highly media-literate reading subjects or whether the interpretive context engineered their criticality; but discussants produced consistently suspicious readings of media-trickery (such as the targeting-practices of media deliberately excluded raced-black parents; or competition between 'media brands' was a money-making racket that produced uncertainty). This criticality about media persuasion did not, on the whole, lead to discussants' outright rejection of the talking-about-sex technology in their parenting practice – this idea is discussed below. This chapter does not imply that any/all readers (and parents) would read didactic texts, nor talk about parenting, in these ways. The point was to unpack appropriation of expertise in *this* interpretive context.

'What is culture?' stories: Modern positions of mobility, hybridity and change

Discussions were characterised by narrative constructions of childhood, childrearing and sexual socialisation – invariably prefaced by the possessive qualifier *'In my culture ...'* – which clearly marked the cultures from which parenting practices evolved. Raced-black, South African women/mothers told stories about traditional *isi-Xhosa* cultural values and practices of family life entrenched in kinship systems within rural settlements or poor communities. These familial practices included, for example, extended networks of child custody; father-absence due to migrant labour or desertion; punitive styles of childrearing that enforced compliance; and customary rules regarding respect for elders that regulated when/how children may interact with their parents, including a 'taboo' on talking about sex. Such stories of traditional African culture/s are familiar in the discourse on 'differences' between groups of people in South Africa, and have long colonial and apartheid genealogies of racialisation, exoticisation and exclusion – as well as appealing to a sense of 'heritage' and 'authentic identity' (Spiegel and Boonzaaier, 1988).

These stories functioned as powerfully acculturated subject positions for speakers in several ways. Firstly, the stories of 'how-it-*still*-is' figured African cultural values and practices around sex, reproduction and children that are recalcitrant to change. South African public health research repeatedly documents how such 'in-my-culture' constructions become 'obstacles' to talking about and changing the sexual risks inherent in patriarchal gender relations, hetero-normative forms of unprotected penetrative sex or childcare arrangements within dispersed families (e.g. LeClerc-Madlala, 2001, 2002; Patton, 1992; Richter, 1994; Walker and Gilbert, 2002). Delius and Glaser (2002) have tracked genealogies of traditional deployments of sex in South Africa to figure a 'cultural system' whose capacity to regulate itself within a heterosexually driven HIV/AIDS epidemic has been 'irrevocably damaged' by Christianised colonisation, apartheid oppression and poverty since the seventeenth century. The 'taboo' on biological parents talking with their children about sex has thus been found as over-determined by *inter alia* limited daily proximity and authoritarian relationships with children, reliance on others and elders for the formal tasks/rituals of sexual socialisation, and belief that sexual instruction of children produces curiosity and experimentation (Kelly and Ntlabati, 2002; Paruk et al., 2005).

Secondly, the authenticity of the traditional African culture narratives afforded raced-black *isiXhosa*-women/mothers powerful positions from which to control how 'culture' was spoken about in group discussions. In Extract 1, Xoliswe's story is told against a raced-white participant's (Ann) attempt to defend the integrity of traditional African cultural systems of sexual socialisation and parenting from the western expertise that inscribes the *Straight Talk* text. Xoliswe's story powerfully articulates her subjection to western sex-communication technologies as a risk deterrent: she unequivocally uses 'these advices' in talking with her own children about sex and risk, and the children she teaches at her school.

Extract 1: Xoliswe's story

Xoliswe: I was myself 16 years *[old]* with a baby there, pregnant there in those rural areas. My son he was born when I was at school because it, that is why I say it ...

Lindy: I think you're telling us that this traditional way of no talking about sex didn't work to protect you from that pregnancy?

Xoliswe: Yes, when I read this *Straight Talk*, I can see these are things that we did not know then, and these things, such talk about love, boys that have electric sex in them *[laughter]*, telling girls their power to get condoms before sex, these things are .... They are better, better than our culture of no talking with kids. I use these advices like this *Straight Talk* when I'm talking to kids, kids at school, my kids, definitely yes I use it ...

Rick: That's the opposite of what Ann was saying just now.

Xoliswe: No, yes, it is true, my people or Xhosa people they say in our culture we do not talk sex and such matters, and this talking these are the ways of whites. This is what they say, eh, I don't know. I don't know what that culture of the Xhosa is now. Is it our Xhosa culture to ... not to educate to our children properly with sex because our parents and ancestors did it? Then the culture stops like that in the olden time when instead it is changing with the modern time in South Africa. That is what I think. I can say they *[our parents]* didn't have AIDS then, they did not have proper education in apartheid, they were poor there in the homelands. It is different times now, we Xhosas do not wear the skins of animals *[laughter]*, you know, women digging fields, sending children to look after some goats *[laughter]*. It must change, so our African culture must learn to talk sex properly like the whites if this can help to save our children.

Ann: Yes, that is different to what I said earlier. I was thinking about keeping local knowledge intact, respecting that protecting what was good in that from this *loveLife* stuff.

Stories of traditional African culture are powerful in such South African group discussions because of the visceral drama and exotic spectacle of their experiences; and because they are inextricably entwined with the oppression and poverty of underdevelopment in colonial- and apartheid-pasts. This elicits uneasiness and guilt in their audience/s, polices culture-talk and positions raced-black subjects as saturated with culture, as *Others*, against raced-white subjects who are figured as 'culture-free' within taken-for-granted as privileged, and therefore unremarkable and unmalleable, subjective practices of living (see Mills, 1997; Stoler, 1995; Swartz, 1998). Xoliswe's story of her own acculturated sex experience in Extract 1 exposes Ann's cultural relativist position (defending African cultural traditions) as naïve, sentimental and patronising. Xoliswe positions herself in this exchange as *cultural spokesperson* or *cultural interpreter* with rights to tell the truth about restrictions and risks inherent in traditional African cultural practices, and to speak *against* her culture. Now a well-educated professional schoolteacher, this carefully wrought middle-classed status permits Xoliswe to adopt positions outside her 'cultural cage', and to engage in more 'liberated', 'modern', 'enlightened', 'western' parenting practices – a conversion she strikingly articulates in racialised terms in Extract 1 as 'talk[ing about] sex properly like the whites'.

Xoliswe's appreciative performance of western expertise in her pedagogisation of sex for/with children does not confirm that she had actually been 'persuaded' to change her childrearing practices as a result of exposure to the rhetoric/messaging of the *Straight Talk* text or similar didactic parenting technologies. Fairclough (1995) makes the useful distinction in positioning related to consumption between *rhetorical persuasion* and *ideological interpellation*. Thus, while reading subjects may dis-identify with the positions/techniques offered them by didactic texts, and not be persuaded by the rhetorical tactics deployed for this purpose, this does *not* mean they escape inscription by, or subjective participation within, dominant discourses of the *psy-complex* or epidemiological risk expertise. This view reiterates Rose's (2007) contention that biological citizens have limited bandwidths for discursive negotiation within hegemonies of expertise. This is evident in Extract 1, where Xoliswe's story powerfully mobilises her own girlhood experience of unwanted pregnancy as definitive proof of the need for change towards a better, healthier lifeworld for children. Thus, Xoliswe finds her 'voice' as a maternal subject and South African, biological citizen – to *talk about* sex with children, to *speak out* about sex against the backwardness and harm of traditional cultural practices – within powerfully emotive discourses of liberation from apartheid, class mobility, modernity and progress. She challenges closed notions of culture through drawing on a *'then-and-now'* genre of story-telling, which starkly establishes the different opportunities and risks of modern life – with concomitant responsibilities inscribed on adult-custodians to 'save our children', presumably from apartheid history, traditional African culture and HIV/AIDS, to fulfil our and their promised/promising future in South Africa (see Posel, 2004).

The references in Extract 1 to '*our* children', as if collectively owned, draw on a *social-ownership-of-children discourse* that powerfully repels the individualisation of maternal, dyadic or nuclear responsibilities usually associated with childrearing practices of the western *psy-complex*, to fabricate a social web of valued relationships, inputs, supports, incentives, resources, systems, policies and rights around developing children (Burman, 2008). The opening out of multiple sites of implantation of sexual knowledge to include siblings, peers, grandparents, teachers and television, calls forth a different kind of parent and styles of relationship and communication between children and their parents. A Foucauldian genealogy of the forms and functioning of families and the custodial responsibilities they prescribe towards children, finds these objects/subjects forged within shifting socio-historical conditions (Rose, 1990). Conditions of sexual risk in an advanced HIV epidemic manufacture children as citizens who are at once sexually knowing *and* vulnerable, and consequently who require – and demand – particular kinds of parenting, monitoring, support and intervention (Singer, 1993). Such shifts are clearly articulated in Nokuthula's narrative of her mothering in Extract 2.

Extract 2: Nokuthula's story

Nokuthula: I think anyway now the pressure is tilting away from us as parents and the values of the home, because our children are now in these multi-racial schools where they learn a lot, even the language that they learn now coming from these schools.

Lindy: *[Pause]* The language they learn, do you mean swearing and dirty stuff for sex?

Nokuthula: No. No I'm saying that they are free now to ask us so many of questions. They are not like the kids in the [*rural Transkei*] villages, who were afraid of asking parents questions, scared of getting punished. Our children, they are not afraid to ask things about sex, or to tell their parents the rules. I have a little girl in Grade 2, I ate a banana one day and threw the skin out the window, and she was furious. She said, 'Why are you littering, we were told at school not to litter, why are you doing that?' And old as I am, I became so ashamed of what I was doing *[laughter]*. The pressure now ... I think the pressure now is they are going to bend our rules, the rules of our culture. We will not be as rigid as before. We cannot be rigid because it will not work with our kids *[laughter]*.

Lindy: Do you think that that's a bad thing *[laughter]*, a good thing?

Nokuthula: It's a good thing, yes, eh, it's good. They ask us as their parents about sex. They watch *Days* and *The Bold* [*soap operas on television*] and she will say, 'Ma, Ridge was doing this and that and so' *[laughter]* and 'What is that thing of kissing?' *[laughter]* I wouldn't do that to my own mother *[laughter]* but she is doing it to me and I don't see anything wrong with it, it's good, it's better like this.

In Extract 2, Nokuthula clearly figures the modern shifts in her mothering praxes in the quality of her 'relationship' with her daughter – different, positively so, to her memory of her relationship with own mother – and in her role as primary sexual socialisation agent. Along the lines of a social-ownership-of-children discourse, raced-black children's sexualised selves are powerfully figured as re-invented, activated and empowered through new educational opportunities in post-apartheid South Africa. This schooling confers a language of citizenship, including sexual citizenship: a young subject who was aware of 'rights' and 'rules' of socially cooperative responsibility; and who is 'free' to ask questions, and *not* bowed by the customary rules of traditional African culture, sex-talk taboo or parental authority/distance. The explicit marking of this schooling as 'multi-racial' in Extract 2 reiterates that raced-black children are rightfully being inscribed with psychology-sanctioned, responsibly middle-classed, sexual subjectivities of 'whiteness', 'citizenship' and 'modernity' denied them in the apartheid-past (cf. Stoler, 1995). The figure of an eight-year-old daughter challenging her mother for littering, or asking about kissing, becomes emblematic of these shifts of relationship, emotional closeness, communication and power, with youthful subjects as *agents* of these changes.

Nokuthula's account of her communication with her daughter in Extract 2 does not accredit any formal sources of didactic parenting technology; it simply 'feels better' than her experience with her own mother, 'right' and 'good'. Nokuthula's conversations with her children appear as (child-initiated) discussions of ordinary events and sexual issues related to watching American soap operas on South African television (*Days of our Lives* and *The Bold and the Beautiful*), in which children may ask, talk back and confront. The form and content of her pedagogical interactions about sex appear as docile subjection within western psychological praxes of child-centred parenting with fearful silences and punishments overwritten by normalisation of everyday conversations about sex, sexuality and risk. However, Nokuthula's sexual citizenship – still within the confines of the western *psy-complex* – is negotiated within wider matrices of modernity that circulate through post-apartheid discourses of education and opportunity and global media cultures.

Different to Xoliswe's earlier call to '*save* our children', with its allusions to rescuing children as innocent victims of history, poverty, culture, sex and risk (see Extract 1), Nokuthula's maternal positioning in Extract 2 is figured as responsive to activated youthful subjects, evident in 'Our children, they are not afraid to ask things about sex, or to tell their parents the rules.' Such a *discourse of youth activism*, of young people leading subjective and social transition, is not of course new in South Africa. Raced-black youth activism mobilised in the struggle against apartheid fashioned much-vaunted 'young lion' and 'warrior' subject positions that were said to have dismantled apartheid schooling and destabilised traditional relations with authoritarian parents in raced-black families (e.g. Campbell, 1997; Dawes, 1994; Stevens and Lockhat, 1997). HIV-prevention campaigning to rekindle such youth-culture activism in order to fabricate sexually knowing, risk-responsible, entrepreneurial and upwardly mobile young citizens – such as by *loveLife* – has met with various resistances, not least being how resource-poor parents are to economically manage, socially support or psychologically engage with such youth subjectivities (LeClerc-Madlala, 2002; Parker, 2003; Posel, 2004; Wilbraham, 2002, 2009).

'Why are you listening to the whites?': Defensive cultural positions

Within a theme of class-mobility aspirations, conversions to western expertise – evident in taking proffered advice on talking to children about sex to inoculate them against risk – were not always a constructive parenting experience for *isiXhosa*-mothers of post-pubertal girls, in particular; situated as they were in communities where traditional cultural sexual norms held sway. While Xoliswe's and Nokuthula's stories (in Extracts 1 and 2) navigated communication about sex with their younger children with confidence, Thandi's narrative account of her mothering 'mistake' in Extract 3 unfolds in relation to her first daughter's unwanted pregnancy. Thandi's continuing story about her second daughter has been cut due to constraints of space in this chapter as has been the interactive positioning as discussants received and responded to her confessions. I note that the discussants and myself as a raced-white researcher constituted other audiences – as assenting and dissenting voices – that placed her mothering decisions under surveillance; as do the readers of this chapter.

Extract 3: Thandi's story

Thandi: I know it is not in the Xhosa way, that cultural custom of my people, the parents do not talk to their children, it is like you *[Nkosi]* said, but this was not the rural areas, but in Mdantsodi where we lived, that is the township nearby Uitenhage. Me and my husband we are educated people, teachers, and when my daughter menstruated, I said to my husband, I will talk to her this and this, because it is dangerous with HIV and pregnancy in this community, such things, and she will be protected with that information. I talked, I told her many many things *[about sex]*, even though my husband said to me, eh, don't do that, you make her want to try that sex.

Lindy: Your husband didn't agree with this or support you?

Thandi: Yes, he is a church-going man, Methodist. Our family is that way, raised in that god-fearing way where sex is for marriage. That is not the Xhosa custom, but it is from the church and the children must know this too. *[Pause]* Ai, she [*Thandi's daughter*] did not listen to anything, nothing that I talked nicely to her, that is how children these days they are very naughty with their parents. She was pregnant when she was Grade 9, 15 years or so. The family of the boy gave money, it was not much but then we sent him [*the baby*] to grandmother, my own mother [*in rural Transkei*] so she [*daughter*] could go to school, but her mind was not there for a long time, her mind was with this boyfriend with a job in town and a car. Afterwards, he went to Joberg, it was a

> disappointment for her but it was better at least with schooling. She is 18 years now, very late for Grade 10, but trying with that again .... [*And a few lines further on*] I know I made a mistake. My people, the community there in Mdantsodi laughed. They said, haai, you are very stupid to be listening to whites, the whites that tell you you must talk about sex, this and that, this and that, this talking sex is white values. It is not of our culture, your husband told you, and now your daughter is pregnant because you did not listen to your husband.

In Extract 3, Thandi positions herself and her husband, as parents, at a nexus of contradictory threads of subjectivity – as 'educated' and 'church-going' people who live in an urban township characterised by hetero-normative sexual culture perceived as 'dangerous' for girls. Several issues leap from this nexus. Decisions about parenting practice – for example, to talk about sex with children or not, how and when – are seldom simple, rational, individual choices produced through being persuaded by an expert technology or being scared by scientific evidence in a didactic text. Spousal disagreement about strategies of talking with children about sex, and management of adolescent sexualised subjectivities in particular, have been widely documented internationally; and it has been argued that such communication and management is taken-for-granted as mothers' work (Burman, 2008). Thus, parenting decisions, and sustained changes of practice, are negotiated in complex, intersectional planes of sight within the domestic cell and the audiences beyond it; constituting layers of surveillance and contradictory voices of history, culture, counsel, experience, judgement and normalisation. In Thandi's tragedy, these inter-texts appear as a Greek Chorus chattering about her hubris and fall: a husband and father of her children; her two adolescent daughters; her own mother; the pastor of her church; various neighbours; schoolteachers at her workplace; her daughter's boyfriend and his family; and 'whites' as unspecified Others outside her community.

The *presence* of talking about sex – rather than qualities and topics of her talk – is taken in Thandi's story as 'choosing' raced-white expertise over local knowledges about risk-avoidance; and she recounts the humiliating failure of her chosen talk-technology (in her 15-year-old daughter's pregnancy). Thandi incurs shame and ridicule within her community for 'listening to the whites', but also for having her middle-classed, raced-white aspirations for her daughters exposed, and for stubbornly ignoring her husband's wishes. In Thandi's inter-textual narrative of the community-audience, she is positioned as 'trying for white' or as that postcolonial sellout, a 'coconut' – black skin with white values inside (Stoler, 1995). Thandi's 'own' voice, which initially adopts western psychological talk-technology (e.g. '*I said* to my husband, *I will talk* to her this and this ...'), is lost within the accusing inter-texts in her narrative in Extract 3; but she later opts for no-talking about sex with her second daughter, realigning herself with traditional cultural custom, and this daughter also becomes pregnant. Taken together, her confessional stories recount her maternal culpability in her daughters' errant experiences of sex and this entrenches her maternal subjection to *psy-complex* logic, most notably that she mistakenly talked about sex *and* mistakenly remained silent, and therefore both daughters became pregnant by *her* mistake (Burman, 1994). This maternal assumption of individual responsibility to 'shape' a daughter in ways that 'conduct her conduct' within wider social and sexual risks (Walkerdine and Lucey, 1989), forms the head/heart of disciplined and risk-vigilant subjectivities of an apparatus of government within a neo-liberal late-capitalist democracy (Rose, 1998). But it implies clashing or deep problematisations of HIV-citizenship sanctioned by the *psy-complex* within developing world conditions, and indeed may only be seen to work effectively where the *psy-complex* enjoys hegemonic status.

Thandi achieves some measure of narrative atonement for her mistaken talking and her first daughter's pregnancy in Extract 3 through positioning herself within a discourse that privileges formal education as the preferred route of social and subjective escape from apartheid's oppression, from culturally entrenched dependence on patriarchs and from poverty. She figures herself and her husband as having succeeded in this class mobility through becoming career professionals through hard work (e.g. 'We are educated people, teachers'), and she is impelled to maintain this class status through inscription of such ethics and values on her children. Her narrative systematically removes the irruptions of her daughter's pregnancy and sexual dalliance with an older/richer boyfriend by getting her schooling back on track.

Conclusion

The Foucauldian approach to didactic health-media discourse as an apparatus of government taken in this chapter examined the operations and effects of expert parenting technologies deployed to prevent risk. Informed by discourses of childrearing within the western *psy-complex*, and powerfully coupled to epidemiological and medical knowledge about sexual risks faced by heterosexually active youth in South Africa, parenting technologies prescribed particular styles and contents of communication about sexuality, sex and sexual issues with children in order to 'risk-proof' them against HIV infection and unwanted pregnancy. This chapter explored the usefulness of such technologies – in terms of dynamics of persuasion, negotiated positioning and appropriative practice in accounts of parenting and biological, sexual and HIV citizenship – to South African, raced-black, *isiXhosa*-speaking, middle-classed schoolteachers/mothers in discussion groups. Predictably, the work of subjectification through expertise was piecemeal, with dispersed intersecting inputs into, different rationales for and voices of commentary on particular childrearing practices (e.g. Hall, 1997; Mills, 1997; Wetherell, 1998). The mothering choices/stories were complexly negotiated within various audiences as communities of practice, regulated by surveillance of norms, and tightly manoeuvred into existing domestic resources and arrangements, and personal experiences and challenges (Kruger, 2006).

This chapter operated within the Foucauldian understanding of 'technology' as the strategic organisation of practices to produce certain outcomes of action, or to direct conduct, in some discursively desirable way (Rose, 1998). Following from Thandi's impotence and uncertainty in Extract 3, 'technology' – or the *techne* (technical operation) of the *psy-complex* – might be pushed in oppositional directions to garner the critical impacts of the analysis in this chapter. Firstly, as a way of *constructively engaging* in this field of HIV prevention, this chapter's ideas might be put to work in improving the effectiveness of the *techne* of parent-pedagogy. Rather than simply suggesting that existing didactic mass media materials, such as *Straight Talk/Lovelines* in *Fairlady*, be tweaked to produce foolproof and failsafe parenting techniques for sex communication with young people, it is recommended that multi-levelled, participatory interventions are added on, providing spaces for contradiction, difference, dialogue, interrogation and re-fabrication of meaningful practice within *and* against existing norms (cf. Campbell, 2003; Patton, 1996). This would involve, for example, breaking down the binary divisions between talk-versus-no-talk, or between western-versus-traditional technologies, to forge alternative practices as hybrids, in between.

Secondly, the epistemological approach adopted in this study provides a critical space to *step back* into; and tools to cut open, reflect on and disengage from western *psy-complex* parenting technologies as the 'talking cure' for the advanced HIV/AIDS epidemic in South Africa. This process crucially rethinks what we think the problem is, takes stock of the knowledge generated as solutions and gathers wits to move on in other ways. For example, what should 'research on HIV/AIDS' – itself a technology that is geared towards risk prevention, reducing stigma, improving treatment and care, honouring life/living – look like, do and be used for? The theoretically positioned, close-grained analytical attention to particular context-contingent inter-subjectivities in this chapter – raced-black, middle-classed South African mothers talking about what they did/do right and wrong with their children – represents an act of resistance, an attempt to 'do' research differently from massively funded, atheoretical, solipsistic, intervention project-work, that is driven to act ever more urgently in global/local epidemics to produce measurable behavioural outcomes.

Finally, why are the individualised parenting technologies of the western *psy-complex* so appealing to (globally funded) South African interventions within risk-infested, impoverished communities? This cuts to critiques of *governmentality* by expertise within New Public Health movements in advanced neo-liberal democracies (Lupton, 1999), that find in the face of collapsing mass mobilisations towards social welfare, individuals are responsibilised through disciplinary power to avoid risk and to carry the consequences as personal liability when things go wrong. Thus, obscuring the obvious economic benefits and risk-safeties of middle-classed communities, the marketing of risk-prevention through a 'proper parenting' technology appeals because, through making mothers responsible for ensuring 'an HIV-free generation', it appears to ward off the catastrophic economic future that is anticipated in an advanced epidemic, with millions of South Africans requiring antiretroviral treatment as a public health benefit, and/or dying of AIDS. Prevention technologies continue to mobilise that spectacle to galvanise docile action towards a myth of HIV-freedom and risk-safety.

Acknowledgements

This chapter was drawn from a wider study on pedagogical materials for parents in HIV/AIDS epidemic in South Africa, and was financially supported by a scholarship from the *National Research Foundation*. I am also grateful to *Fairlady* magazine for permission to use the *Lovelines* texts and to the discussants for sharing their parenting stories. Earlier/other versions of this chapter were presented at the *British Sociological Association Conference*, University of East London, UK, 12–14 April 2007; and published in *African Journal of AIDS Research*, 2008, 7, 1, 95–109.

References

Alldred, P. (1996) 'Whose expertise? Conceptualizing resistance to advice about childrearing' in E. Burman, G. Aitken, P. Alldred, R. Allwood, T. Billington, B. Goldberg, A. Gordo Lopez, C. Heenan, D. Marks and S. Warner (eds), *Psychology discourse practice: from regulation to resistance* (London: Taylor and Francis).

Bhana, A., Petersen, I., Mason, A., Mahintsho, Z., Bell, C. and McKay, M. (2004) 'Children and youth at risk: adaptation and pilot study of CHAMP (AmaQhawe) programme in South Africa', *African Journal of AIDS Research*, 3, 1, 33–41.

Blackman, L. and Walkerdine, V. (2001) *Mass hysteria: critical psychology and media studies* (Basingstoke: Palgrave Macmillan).

Blake, S., Simkin, L., Ledsky, R., Perkins, C. and Calabrese, J. (2001) 'Effects of parent–child communications interventions on young adolescents' risk for early onset of sexual intercourse', *Family Planning Perspectives*, 33, 2, 52–67.

Burman, E. (1994) *Deconstructing developmental psychology* (London: Routledge).

—— (2008) *Developments: child, image, nation* (London: Routledge).

Campbell, C. (1997) 'Self-esteem in context: A case study of the motivational processes underlying social identity construction by township youth', *Psychology in Society*, 22, 20–36.

—— (2003) *'Letting them die': how HIV/AIDS prevention programmes often fail* (Oxford: The International African Institute, with James Curry).

Dawes, A. (1994) 'The emotional impact of political violence' in A. Dawes and D. Donald (eds), *Childhood and adversity: psychological perspectives from South African research* (Cape Town: David Philip).

Dawes, A. and Donald, D. (1994) 'Understanding the psychological consequences of adversity' in A. Dawes and D. Donald (eds), *Childhood and adversity: psychological perspectives from South African research* (Cape Town: David Philip).

Dean, M. (1994) 'A social structure of many souls: moral regulation, government and self-regulation', *Canadian Journal of Sociology*, 19, 145–68.

Delius, P. and Glaser, C. (2002) 'Sexual socialization in South Africa: an historical perspective', *African Studies*, 61, 27–54.

Fairclough, N. (1992) *Discourse and social change* (Cambridge: Polity Press).

—— (1995) *Media discourse* (London: Edward Arnold).

Foster, G., Levine, C. and Williamson, J. (eds) (2005) *A generation at risk: the global impact of HIV/AIDS on orphans and vulnerable children* (New York: Cambridge University Press).

Foucault, M. (1978) *The history of sexuality, volume 1: an introduction* (Harmondsworth: Penguin).

Grunseit, A., Kippax, S., Aggleton, P., Baldo, M. and Slutkin, G. (1997) 'Sexuality education and young people's sexual behaviour', *Journal of Adolescent Research*, 12, 421–53.

Hall, S. (1997) 'The work of representation', in S. Hall (ed.), *Representation: cultural representations and signifying practices* (London: Sage and Open University Press).

Hermes, J. (1995) *Reading women's magazines: An analysis of everyday media use* (Cambridge: Polity Press).

Kelly, K. and Ntlabati, P. (2002) 'Early adolescent sex in South Africa: HIV interventions and challenges', *Social Dynamics*, 28, 42–63.

Kelly, K., Parker, W. and Oyosi, S. (2001) *Pathways to action: HIV/AIDS prevention, children and young people in South Africa – a literature review* (Johannesburg: Centre for AIDS Development, Research and Evaluation (CADRE)), report commissioned by Save the Children Fund, UK, http://www.cadre.org.za.

Kruger, L. M. (2006) 'Motherhood', in T. Shefer, F. Boonzaaier and P. Kiguwa (eds), *The gender of psychology* (Cape Town: UCT Press).

LeClerc-Madlala, S. (2001) 'Demonizing women in the era of AIDS: on the relationships between cultural constructions of both HIV/AIDS and femininity', *Society in Transition*, 32, 38–46.

—— (2002) 'Youth, HIV/AIDS and the importance of sexual culture and context', *Social Dynamics*, 28, 20–41.

loveLife (2000a) *Love them enough to talk about sex* (Johannesburg: *loveLife*) http://www.lovelife.org.za/parents.

—— (2000b) *Talking and listening: parents and teenagers together – find out how to make it easier* (Johannesburg: *loveLife*) http://www.lovelife.org.za/parents.

Lupton, D. (1999) *Risk* (London: Routledge).

Lupton, D. and Tulloch, J. (1998) 'The adolescent "unfinished body": reflexivity and HIV/AIDS risk', *Body and Society*, 4, 2, 19–34.

McQuail, D. (1994) *Mass communication theory: an introduction, 3rd edition* (London: Sage).

Miller, D., Kitzinger, J., Williams, K. and Beharrell, P. (1998) *The circuit of mass communication: media strategies, representation and audience reception in the AIDS crisis* (London: Sage).

Mills, S. (1994) 'Introduction', in S. Mills (ed.), *Gendering the reader* (Hemel Hempstead: Harvester Wheatsheaf).

—— (1997) *Discourse* (London: Routledge).

Parker, I. (1992) *Discourse dynamics: critical analysis for social and individual psychology* (London: Routledge).

Parker, W. (2003) *Re-appraising youth prevention in South Africa: the case of loveLife*, paper presented at International AIDS Conference, Durban, 3–6 August, http://www.cadre.org.za.

Paruk, Z., Petersen, I., Bhana, A., Bell, C. and McKay, M. (2005) 'Containment and contagion: how to strengthen families to support youth HIV-prevention in South Africa', *African Journal of AIDS Research*, 4, 1, 57–63.

Patton, C. (1992) 'From nation to family: containing African AIDS', in A. Parker, M. Russo, D. Summer and P. Yaeger (eds), *Nationalisms and sexualities* (New York: Routledge).

—— (1996) *Fatal advice: How safe-sex education went wrong* (Durham: Duke University Press).

Posel, D. (2004) 'Getting the nation talking about sex: reflections on the discursive constitution of sexuality in South Africa since 1994', *Agenda*, 62, 52–63.

Richter, L. (1994) 'Economic stress and its influence on the family and caretaking patterns', in A. Dawes and D. Donald (eds), *Childhood and adversity: psychological perspectives from South African research* (Cape Town: David Philip).

Rose, N. (1990) *Governing the soul: the shaping of the private self* (London: Routledge).

—— (1992) 'Engineering the human soul: analyzing psychological expertise', *Science in Context*, 5, 351–69.

—— (1998) *Inventing our selves: psychology, power and personhood* (Cambridge: Cambridge University Press).

—— (2007) *The politics of life itself: biomedicine, power and subjectivity in the 21st century* (Princeton, NJ: Princeton University Press).

Singer, L. (1993) *Erotic welfare: sexual theory and politics in the age of epidemic* (London: Routledge).

Spiegel, A. and Boonzaier, E. (1988) 'Promoting tradition: images of the South African past', in E. Boonzaier and J. Sharp (eds), *South African keywords: the uses and abuses of political concepts* (Cape Town: David Philip).

Stainton-Rogers, R. and Stainton-Rogers, W. (1992) *Stories of childhoods: shifting agendas of child concern* (Hemel Hempstead: Harvester Wheatsheaf).

Stevens, G. and Lockhat, R. (1997) 'Coca-cola kids: Reflections on black adolescent identity development in post-apartheid South Africa', *South African Journal of Psychology*, 27, 250–7.

Stoler, A. L. (1995) *Race and the education of desire: Foucault's history of sexuality and the colonial order of things* (Durham: Duke University Press).

Swartz, L. (1998) *Culture and mental health: a southern African view* (Cape Town: Oxford University Press).

Thomas, K. (2004) 'A better life for some: The *loveLife* campaign and HIV/AIDS in South Africa', *Agenda*, 62, 28–35.

Walker, L. and Gilbert, L. (2002) 'HIV/AIDS: South African women at risk', *African Journal of AIDS Research*, 1, 1, 75–85.

Walkerdine, V. and Lucey, H. (1989) *Democracy in the kitchen: regulating mothers and socialising daughters* (London: Virago).

Wetherell, M. (1998) 'Positioning and interpretative repertoires: conversation analysis and post-structuralism in dialogue', *Discourse and Society*, 9, 387–412.

Wilbraham, L. (2002) 'Parents talking with youth about sex and AIDS: Some problems with health education materials', *AIDS Bulletin*, 11, 4, 6–9.

—— (2004) 'Discursive practice: Analyzing a *Lovelines* text on sex communication for parents', in D. Hook (ed.), *Critical psychology* (Landsdowne, Cape Town: UCT Press).

—— (2008) 'Parental communication with children about sex in the HIV/AIDS epidemic in South Africa: gendered, raced, classed and cultural appropriations of *Lovelines*', *African Journal of AIDS Research*, 7, 1, 95–109.

—— (2009) 'Manufacturing willingness: Parents and young people talking about sex in a HIV & AIDS epidemic in South Africa', *South African Journal of Psychology*, 39, 1, 59–74.

Wilton, T. (1997) *EnGendering AIDS: deconstructing sex, text and epidemic* (London: Sage).

6
HIV Transitions: Consequences for Self in an Era of Medicalisation

Paul Flowers

Introduction

In the West the normalisation of HIV has crystallised a singular, dominant, medical construction of HIV infection. Of course medical constructions of HIV have always been present and central to understanding HIV, yet recently, in conjunction with the advent of antiretroviral therapy (ART), they have become far more salient. This chapter, with an exploration of the experiences of people living with HIV in the UK, seeks to refocus the reader upon a range of psychosocial issues which can sometimes be overlooked, or overshadowed, when faced with the brightness and clarity of the biomedical narrative of HIV. Through drawing on a range of positive people's experiences the chapter tentatively explores how processes of HIV normalisation rely upon the medicalisation of HIV and a concomitant process of the minimisation of psychosocial issues. In the global context of difficulties accessing treatments and care, these psychosocial concerns may indeed appear minor, yet sometimes, and often in surprising ways, the biomedical depends upon the psychosocial to function.

Medical constructions increasingly dominate other key ways of thinking about HIV, perhaps in ways which are not always helpful. Such a model, for example, highlights the centrality of a medical model of living with HIV, in which 'health' is measured in primarily biomedical terms (for example CD4 and Viral load) and other 'softer' understandings, such as quality of life or measures of psychosocial distress appear as less important. In the West, organisations for people living with HIV have dwindled and in the UK activism has all but disappeared. Even HIV prevention, and the concomitant drive to change people's behaviour through an understanding of sexual conduct and its social determinants, is being replaced by ideas of addressing 'onwards transmission' through biomedical means. Circumcision is being promoted as a means of prevention, for example (see Katz and Wright, 2008). Equally, HIV testing is increasingly seen as pivotal to HIV prevention, despite a lack of convincing evidence showing any clear patterns in terms of corresponding changes towards reductions in HIV risk related behaviour. HIV testing can only relate to prevention through biomedical means, through reducing population viraemia through early diagnosis and ensuring all positive people are on medication with reduced levels of viral load in the bodies. The messy complexities of addressing people in a holistic sense, with their social interactions and meaning-laden sexual conduct seems a far less attractive, less measurable and increasingly arduous, and unrelentingly political, option for policy makers and government alike.

It could be argued that, whereas in the past, the unimpeded action of virus facilitated a host of psychological and sociocultural understandings and responses to HIV, the effective action of medication upon the virus has rendered the positive body as mere 'setting' for action. Critically, within these kinds of construction, the HIV positive person is reduced to a disease vector within prevention, and adherence and the work of managing side effects becomes relevant only as the mechanism by which the medication can work its wonders.

In contrast to the coalescence of an increasingly singular and biomedical model of HIV at least in affluent countries, there has been a diversification and arguably a relegation of both psychosocial and sociocultural constructions of living with HIV. These latter understandings of HIV have not simply withered, or atrophied, but have become increasingly dissipated and easily dismissed. The global impact of HIV, with all its stark inequalities, and the often awkward and profound differences in poverty and wider political and social circumstances, means that the apparent universality of the biomedical offers a particularly palatable way of engaging with the global epidemic. Treichler's work regarding an 'epidemic of signification' (Treichler, 1987) still aptly captures the range of sociocultural responses to HIV although perhaps now, more than ever, some understandings dominate and overshadow others. This chapter explores some of these, now 'secondary', psychosocial constructions of living with HIV through drawing upon a series of experiential studies which sought to explore the experience of living with HIV in the twenty-first century.

As a rich developed country, the UK is fortunate to have a mostly effective health care structure which enables the majority of HIV positive people to access HIV treatment and care, for free, from the point of diagnosis. In a review of the impact of ART upon the psychosocial and health care needs of positive people in the UK, Green and Smith (2004) illustrate how the 'normalisation' of HIV (DeCock and Johnson, 1998) has led to the transformation of HIV from fatal disease to a chronic manageable infection. The main premise of their review was to chart the changes which have occurred in the UK in the wake of effective treatment for HIV. They note that, overall, the psychosocial needs of positive people living in the UK in the post-ART era are now much more focussed upon the 'everyday' problems of 'living with HIV' rather than the difficulties of disease, dying and death. Similarly, Siegel and Lekas (2002), in a recent international review, focus on the idea of changes in psychosocial and social issues since the introduction of ART. They conclude that for people living with HIV where treatments are available, 'there are many continuities as well as discontinuities in the experience of living with HIV/AIDS over the last two decades' (page S74). In terms of discontinuities in the experience of living with HIV, the health benefits of ART are clear: reduced morbidity and reduced mortality (Gulick et al., 2003; Kaufmann et al., 2003; Garcia et al., 2004). However, there have been changes in terms of the emergence of new uncertainties, for example, potential longevity instead of almost certain death, the challenges of returning to the workplace, the problems of the potential loss of benefits when health is regained and facing an unanticipated future (Brashers et al., 1999). Equally, there are dilemmas for many positive people in terms of re-engaging with the possibilities of relationships and a reinvigorated interest in sex. Moreover, the side effects of medication bring further psychological challenges, for example, the impact of lipidystrophy (Blanch et al, 2002; Collins et al., 2000). In terms of the continuities in living with HIV, little has changed, for example, Siegel and Lekas (2002) reviewed the literature with regard to assessing the impact of ART upon psychological distress among positive people and found inconclusive evidence. Their review shows no clear relationship between the introduction of ART and either increasing or decreasing distress associated with living with HIV. Similarly, Ciesla and Roberts (2001), in a meta-analytic review of the literature relating to HIV status and depression, report that when comparing HIV positive participants to HIV negative participants, the frequency of a major depressive disorder was two times higher among positive people. This chapter begins to address these 'every day problems' through the presentation of an analysis of interview-based data.

The chapter draws upon data from two studies concerning the experience of living with HIV conducted in the UK between 2001 and 2006. Both studies employed Interpretative Phenomenological Analysis (IPA) which is a qualitative approach that structures data collection and data analysis with a mixture of idiography and hermeneutic phenomenology (for more detail on this approach, see Smith et al., 2009). The studies I will refer to are an Economic and Social Research Council (ESRC) funded project entitled 'Transitions in HIV management', and a small charity project entitled 'The Connected Study' which examined relationships among HIV positive gay men in the post-ART era. The first study sought a diverse sample of positive people from both Glasgow (Scotland) and London (England). It included both gay men and black Africans living in the UK (the two main groups of people affected by HIV in the UK). The 'Connected' study sampled diverse gay and bisexual men living with HIV from across Scotland, mainly from the large urban centres where the HIV epidemic is focused. These studies each had their own particular focus and analytic slant, the transitions study focusing upon the impact of ART and the 'Connected study' focusing upon relational aspects of living with HIV. Yet in this chapter the two studies are fractured and amalgamated to produce an overarching narrative that focuses on the commonality between the two projects. This analysis was structured around four themes: (1) the contingent impact of HIV diagnosis: the past, the future and on-going uncertainty, (2) identity work, loss of self, viral identities, (3) disclosure stories: externalising ambivalent and viral identities and (4) disclosure stories: externalising HIV and identity 'leakage'.

The contingent impact of HIV diagnosis: The past, the future and ongoing uncertainty

The analysis begins with a theme which illustrates the limitations of biomedical constructions of health and HIV. The participants, all with good CD4 counts and thus good apparent health, describe the disparity between their mental and physical health. Their psychological distress relates to the uncertain meaning of their biomedical diagnosis. In the extracts that follow, a sense of the enduring psychological distress associated with HIV emerges. As the literature would suggest, distress relates in part to diagnosis itself (see, for example, Kalichman and Sikkema, 1994) but, in addition, it also relates to what could be described as 'ontological uncertainty'. People diagnosed with HIV often talk of their particular search for meaning, directly in terms of the actual process of diagnosis (what does HIV mean to me now?) but also in terms of the challenges of living well with HIV (adjusting their wider life expectations and sense of mortality). As we see below, behind the self-referent identity work the participants describe, there is a sense of psychological distress that seems to run in parallel with a search for meaning in relation to HIV diagnosis. For many people diagnosed when well, while everything has changed, nothing has changed. Given the context of 'medicalisation', somewhat ironically, in the absence of disease, or the physical manifestation of the virus, people seem to sometimes focus on the internal, or 'psychological'. As Molly suggests:

> Just cause of the results something had actually changed on my face and everything, I think the only thing that happened was emotionally yes, I was really, really, you know injured, but physically nothing changed I had this, I was still in the same state even though I was I think a couple of weeks after my diagnosis, I didn't lose weight I didn't gain weight I didn't, stop dressing the way I did, so, it was quite scary. (Molly, African woman, London)

Molly outlines the expectation of change and a sense of anticipated immediate impact. However, she contrasts this with a sense of how nothing external actually changed. For other African participants, like Rachel, the meaning of diagnosis was intricately bound to her personal biography and experiences of AIDS in Africa.

> Respondent: I think for me, I just felt my life was gone, as a youth, as a young woman aspiring for so much in life. I thought that was the end of it. At that time, when I was diagnosed, I wasn't the type who was into make-up at all. That day, I bought ... I used to buy make-up and keep it in my drawers. I got home and all night that's what I was doing.
>
> Interviewer: Doing your face up?
>
> R: Doing my face up, putting all the foundation and doing my face up! I felt I was denied life. I felt I'd never have a child, never have a family, I'd never get married, and I'd never fulfil my career or education prospects. My life was gone, and the way it was handled, the stigma around at the time, the death threats – coming from Africa, I'd seen so many people dying that to me that was the end of my life actually. Yeah. (Rachel, African woman, London)

Rachel's extract details her feelings about the loss of an anticipated future and a wide range of threats of life plans. Her deliberate and focused 'make over' can be understood not only as reflecting the severity of the threat to her identity, but also as an expression of her sudden and enforced living within the present. The temporal horizon associated with her imagined health trajectory had shifted radically. In contrast to Rachel's African experiences, for Scottish gay men like Alex, the efficacy of Western medicine and ART was often cautiously embraced. Yet the history of HIV and concomitant representations of gay men and AIDS remained salient.

> It's a really bizarre process to go through because, you don't really know how to feel, because you're getting all these mixed messages about all the eighties media stuff thing, thinking: well that's it that's my life over; but on the other hand there's all the optimistic stuff around having a long fulfilled life in front of you, so you're trying to balance all that, so what ends up is you're, this totally new identity. (Alex, gay man, Glasgow)

Alex appears caught between the differing constructions of HIV. The present seems constrained by both negative 'ghosts' of the past but also 'positive' anticipations of the future. Alex stresses the effort and work of addressing these potential consequences. Throughout these accounts there tends to be confusion and uncertainty regarding the personal implications of HIV diagnosis, yet there is a powerful and persistent sense of HIV diagnosis having consequences, potentially for health but definitely for self and 'identity'. It is the chronicity of this 'everyday' problem that demands some recognition from service providers and policy makers. Although enduring ontological uncertainty will not kill someone, it does appear to be a source of concern and distress for the research participants. The imposition of the undeniable medical 'truth' of HIV diagnosis and the attendant constellation of ambiguous and contingent meanings consistently led to often profound psychological distress and often marked social withdrawal. It is this inward turn, to what could be described as the management of self, which the next theme addresses more fully.

Identity work, loss of self, viral identities

Although HIV has always been understood as a 'master status' because of the multiple stigmas it engenders, in an era in which, for some, HIV is treatable and in which medical discourse focuses upon its 'normalisation', it may seem surprising that HIV diagnosis still brings with it grave consequences, for self and/or for identity. Pre-ART work highlighted the importance of HIV for self and identity (see, for example, Tewksbury and McGaughey, 1998). Roth and Nelson (1994), for example, charted the production of an identity through the process of HIV diagnosis. They state that receiving an HIV-positive diagnosis was a life-changing event. They described a process of 'becoming an HIV positive self' and note that 'regardless of the way in which the diagnosis is constructed, the patient is still being initiated into a new self, a self that is HIV-positive – a self that many would prefer not to be' (p. 178). The identity talk and identity work, which runs throughout most interviews concerned with living with HIV, speaks volumes about the productive power of biomedicine. In other words, a diagnostic medical process can be pivotal in creating and shaping a sense of self or identity. The rhetoric of HIV normalisation minimises these psychosocial aspects of HIV. It stresses the 'routine' and treatable nature of HIV necessarily without invoking any consequences to self and identity. Its proponents demand an end to 'AIDS exceptionalism' and focus upon the straightforward medical trajectory of testing and treatment. Yet participants battle with their HIV self or HIV identity; the diagnostic category shatters and replaces their previous understandings of self. Yet the mechanics of this agency, or its constructive capacity, are not straightforward, or indeed clear cut. The very fact that HIV resists 'normalisation' and, even where treatments are available, continues to violate sense of self, highlights the centrality and durability of particularly 'social' constructions of HIV. These psychosocial and sociocultural constructions are precisely what HIV normalisation seems to dismiss. The extract from Denis, below, highlights this paradox.

R: I grieved first of all, I had a period of grief, because it was just as if I'd suffered a loss, a loss a part of me had died I think,
I: So when you said: grief and mourning, what were you grieving?
R: It was, it's hard to, to describe, but I just felt as if part of me died, um .... I don't know what that was.
I: You said it's hard to describe it, but have a go ...
R: I don't know, maybe a kind of loss of innocence, ... and the fact that I was going to have to, this was going to be such a major event, something that's going to be hanging over me and that I'm going to have to deal with in almost everything I do every day, which it is. Every morning I woke up I thought oh ... I'd wake up

and think: oh it's a nice day, oh my god I'm HIV positive and I would be down again

I: So you said about the sense of, the sense of grief was the word you used about the loss of ... innocence, a sense of expecting ... well you said about waking up in the morning it's a beautiful day and then ....

R: Yeah it's feeling unhappy that I was, had this horrible thing that was hanging over me that I was very different, had this like big label on my forehead.

I: What do you mean by that?

R: A sort of biohazard symbol, you know, like I'm dangerous, I'm different, that's how it felt, I felt very isolated because of a sort of clinical condition. (Denis, gay man, Scotland)

Denis's 'superficial' language, of 'labels' and 'symbols', and the corresponding sense of personal reduction and transformation, is contrasted with the emotive descriptions of an internal and hidden mental world. While the former does resonate with the rhetoric of normalisation (though clearly, a biohazard symbol is more than a neutral biomedical label), as a mere description of a diagnostic category, the idea of 'HIV as just another disease', it also highlights the centrality of risk: the omnipresence of the uninfected onlooker, the HIV negative person who should take heed of the warning label. These descriptions of psychological distress, particularly when focussed on highlighting isolation, social withdrawal and an emerging dissonance between 'private' and 'public' selves, almost always emphasise the centrality of the 'other'. They embody HIV related stigma as 'felt' rather than 'enacted' (Scambler, 1998). In other words, they highlight how important it is to acknowledge how someone's expectations and assumptions of stigma are as important as social experiences of stigma and discrimination. The multi-leveled extract from Jack illustrates that this choreography of self-presentation is not without its costs.

I think that was really because I had, I just I just didn't know who ... in lots of ways I didn't know who I was, at that time, in the early days of being diagnosed and coming to terms with it, I couldn't stop thinking about it and um ... I had to go through a process of finding out or finding myself again, um, and whilst I was around people that knew me well, I found it really, really exhausting because, well maybe they couldn't tell but I, I was sure, I was paranoid that that they would know that something was wrong, so I was constantly

> trying to be as near to how I imagined myself to being without HIV so ... that in itself made it even more impossible, because the more you try to stop thinking about something, then the harder it becomes, you know so .... (Jack, gay man, Edinburgh)

These extracts show the impact of HIV diagnosis upon ideas of the self, or identity. The two examples both relate to Scottish gay men diagnosed in the twenty-first century who can anticipate access to ART and positive health consequences. The reader may be struck by their similarity with earlier accounts within the history of the epidemic; in terms of self and identity, little has changed (Pierret, 2001; Ezzy, 2000). The psychosocial consequences of HIV diagnosis seem resistant to processes of normalisation. The identity imperative has remained unchanged despite the radical shift in morbidity and mortality that ART has wrought. Although the focus of the extracts presented within this section is clearly upon the internal world of the participant and their adjustment to HIV diagnosis, they also highlight the importance of relational aspects of identity. The following section explores and expands this idea further.

Disclosure stories: Externalising ambivalent and viral identities

The public health imperative to reduce HIV transmission has constructed the issue of HIV status disclosure as a part of safer sex and less often as a means of thinking about access to social support. Here, however, HIV status is presented as an issue firmly related to issues of self and identity. An extract from Lizzy introduces the critical importance of status disclosure. This importance does not relate to health care, public health or reducing transmission, but relates to disclosure as an act of externalising some of the often troubled identity work illustrated in previous sections. She hints at the impact of her status disclosure upon her family and the resulting identity 'work' this has necessitated. Again we see the impact of HIV status as a kind of master status; the 'viral identity' is reorganising her family's perceptions of her.

> I've had to sort of re-build my relationships with my family, sort of from scratch, because I think whatever my family ever thought of me before, I'm not too sure about any more. I don't know whether it's a lack of confidence in myself or a lack of trust in them on my part, I don't know. It's not anything that they do or say but it's what I feel,

> you know. I'm very cautious about everything I do. I'm very cautious about what I say. (Lizzy, African woman, London)

Lizzy's identity seems fragile and she, like Jack above, describes a process of self-monitoring and quite self-conscious self-presentation. Implicitly, HIV diagnosis has erased an identity that had endured many years of family relationships. Similarly, the extract below from Luke emphasises just how high the stakes can be in terms of understanding HIV status disclosure. Luke was a gay man diagnosed when very ill in hospital with HIV-related illness. The extract focuses upon the family once more, perhaps as a fundamental site in which identity, or sense of self, is forged. For Luke, rejection from his children would have meant the loss of his own will to live.

> My younger son he actually went and asked the doctor what was wrong with his dad. He wanted to know why his dad was still in this hospital, why has he got drips, why was there this and ... I said to the doctor 'You can tell him.' I thought, if they reject me I'll just, didn't want to live, but no they went the opposite way. [...] Yeah, but I thought I have to, I'm their dad, I'm someone they look up to [mm] I'm, I'm their mentor. I lost my dad when I was twelve and I thought I've got to be strong for them, and see when I told them I thought, they both cried, we all cried and I thought, I'm not I can't leave you now, I've got to keep well. (Luke, gay man, Edinburgh)

For most participants most of the time, there was a degree of choice, or an understanding of agency, surrounding the issue of status disclosure. However, within many interviews there were added complications in managing others' knowledge of status in terms of issues such as explaining hospital visits and, for those on medication, hiding tablets or taking them in secret. In addition there were challenges relating to explaining periodic illness to friends, family and work colleagues. Keeping secrets added a further dimension of stress and worry to some positive people's lives. It seems a welcome burden that decisions around status disclosure must now be managed, and are now sometimes afforded a sense of choice, rather than being an inevitable event necessitated through death and dying.

Disclosure stories: Externalising HIV and identity leakage

The preceding section outlined how disclosure of HIV antibody status was sometimes problematic partly because of the identity repercussions which followed. This theme explores disclosure further; however it focuses upon the issue of unintentional disclosure. Terry for example, another participant diagnosed with HIV when hospitalised with HIV-related illness, left hospital after losing weight. In an extract reminiscent of other 'healthy' participants' concerns about the salience of their diagnosis to imagined others, when Terry went out to the gay scene, he felt people were accurately 'reading' his HIV status.

R: I suppose when I the first diagnosed and I went out to the bars for the first time it was kind of scary.
I: Why was it scary?
R: Oh you think you've got a big label on you and you're thinner and you think it's obvious. (Terry, gay man, Glasgow)

Once more the metaphor of the label is invoked and the presence of the onlooker is felt. 'Felt' stigma is embodied, the ambiguous symptoms of weight loss are reconstructed as a definitive proof of positive HIV status. The social leakage of HIV status and thus the unintentional disclosure of positive HIV status was a particular concern and not limited to the visible impact of the virus on the body. For some positive people, the side effects of medication rather than the effects of the virus itself are the focus of concern about identity leakage. It seems a frightful irony that in fighting the virus, to resist the ultimate power of the virus to take life and claim the body, the body may still be transformed and appropriated by the effects of medication taken to manage the virus. The redistribution of body fat as a result of ART represents one such arena. As such, in the extract below, Dora an African woman living in London introduces the issue of lipidystrophy.

R: Lipidystrophy ... I think for me that has been my main side effect, the others aren't too bad ... and the skin, the skin rash and all. Other than those two, I feel great around the drugs, but it's the thought of the future.
I: You mentioned lipidystrophy – what is that?
R: Well, some of the drugs lead to body fat changes and the fats lodge in areas of the body other than the others and especially my limbs they go really thin. You've got more muscles, your stomach will go big, you'll get a buffalo hump on your neck. If it's a woman, your bust will get big. Even some men become busty. Those are physical side effects that are so obvious to a number of people that there must be something wrong with you, and even to you yourself,

> especially when it comes to your femininity – when you look at all those body shape changes on you. You can't wear a short skirt anymore, you can't wear a dress because you look like a box or you look like Humpty Dumpty. So there are limitations on what you can do and it's those things that can be very depressive and can make people lose their self-esteem and even decide not to take their medication. (Dora, HIV positive, London)

Dora highlights an additional, and literal, example of the productive, or constitutive capacity of ART to construct HIV positive people. Changes in body shape constrain and limit gender appropriate appearances and can be read by onlookers as signifiers of positive status. Although many people living with HIV have no visible indication of their HIV status, a substantial minority have either facial and/or bodily lipidystrophy. In the quote below Andy talks in detail about his experience of lipidystrophy and illustrates its relevance to the issues of viral identity and disclosure.

> R: I was like, wouldn't come out my house, because to me it was so evident, what I had, even though it wouldn't be evident other people, in my head, if they looked at me, I would direct everything to that place where I had lipidystrophy and turn everything round to having lipidystrophy. So, lipidystrophy ruled my world at that point.
>
> I: What was it about the lipidystrophy that was worrying you?
>
> R: Just because it was HIV. If I had looked like this normally, I wouldn't give a shit. Everything's to do with HIV.
>
> I: Can you explain again. How is it .... Why did it bother you?
>
> R: How do you mean, why did it bother me? Why would it bother you if you were deformed? Through something which you wanted to hide from everybody? Isn't that kind of stating the obvious? Obviously, if you've got something to hide, and you're wearing it on a badge, and that badge can only be read by certain people, it's going to bother you. You know, and if you're somebody who analyses things to death, obviously you're going to analyse the whole situation ... and it's just going to drive you nuts. So the only way to get away from that, is by not exposing yourself to people and viewing yourself, for your own mental ... I mean we could go into so many areas, but for your own mental stability, like when you look at yourself in the mirror, you make sure you face the mirror at a certain angle, so when you look in the mirror,

> everybody puts an expression on their face so that they make themselves look better, so, in the way they want to project themselves, how they think they look because nobody really knows how they look to themselves, and how other people, how you really look. So, obviously your whole life is generated and I knew times of the day when I'd look better than others, so I make sure that I only looked at myself during those times. You know, I'd wear sunglasses all the time because sunglasses take away from the aggressive nature of the look. So, yeah, my whole life at that point, was geared round to not looking like I had lipidystrophy. Plus, I was extremely uncomfortable, I had no fat on the bottom of my feet, I had no fat on my arse, in my knees, you know, so I couldn't walk on wooden floors. (Andy, gay man Edinburgh)

This extract highlights the distress and anxiety that lipidystrophy can cause. Although Andy described the physical pain associated with the condition, there is also a sense of the psychological pain the condition caused (particularly his facial disfigurement). For Andy there were clear concerns relating to the fact he no longer looked like himself and in fact that he looked like a person with HIV. He outlines a distressing physical corollary of the identity dissonance and identity management outlined earlier in this chapter. Moreover he outlines some very real concerns about non-intentional status disclosure. People could 'read' his HIV status without his consent, stripping away any sense of control over this important issue and exposing him to HIV related stigma. The following quote neatly summarises many of the points raised in this section:

> I've seen people get better. I've seen people get better. I mean the pros are more than the cons I think. Speaking from a woman's point of view, I've seen what they've done to some of my friends. You know the way a woman moves, a woman is proud of the way she looks, you know a small waist, nice bum, nice legs and suddenly that's all taken away from you. And in a case where you haven't disclosed your status and people start seeing the body changing – that alone is enough to disclose your status. The practical issues around taking medication, how many times a day, you know, the restrictions, are for someone who hasn't disclosed their status who is in a relationship, when do you take your medication? Do you wait for a partner to go to your bathroom? What happens if you go away for a weekend? What happens if you're working for instance and you have to take your medication at lunchtime and your colleagues are there?

> Someone was telling me about a story where two girls went to ... two young ladies went to a party and eight o'clock is the time when she should take her evening dose. She took her tablets out and was just about to swallow them, when the other friend said 'oh what's that?' She didn't know that the other one was positive. And she said 'oh my headache tablets.' 'Oh, I have a headache too. Can I have some?' What do you do then? You know. (Jessica, African woman, London)

For one African participant, although not having natural childbirth did not present a particular problem in terms of HIV status, the idea of not breastfeeding (and its association with positive HIV status) brought some concerns. As Sarah says:

> R: Not breast feeding. Now that's another thing – breast feeding. I might become, in my culture you breastfeed, it's the best ... I know it's the best thing for the baby, but in this situation it's not going to be. I don't know how my family is going to take that me not feeding.
>
> I: Mm, yeah, I heard a paediatrician actually say that that some of his patients, African women, that the hardest thing for them is not being able to breastfeed because then ...
>
> R: Everything else is not so ... you know, having the caesarean section you can, you can, you can have an explanation for it, but not breast feeding. What explanation do you have? [...] Yeah it is difficult to begin with, but that is the most difficult thing, I don't know how I'm going to tackle that one. Is not breastfeeding. [...] Definitely my mum is going to be .... 'Because you know, you are spending more money buying milk, you know, money you don't have.' That's the most difficult situation. Having the caesarean section I'm not even worried about. Because one in four women nowadays have caesarean sections.
>
> I: It seems it requires some stories, the breast-feeding thing?
>
> R: Yeah, yeah. And also having a sister who has only had a child [that lives with her], not very long ago and she is breastfeeding. She is breastfeeding, for a year, you know. And I look after her and her baby. (Sarah)

Once more it is interesting to note how observable behaviour which may have many potential causal explanations is seen through one particular frame, the leakage of HIV status. 'Felt' stigma emerges once more as having a central role within the work of living with HIV. Critically,

HIV stigma does not seem to have reduced as a result of the widespread availability of ART within the UK. HIV stigma is core to the management of an HIV identity. The normalisation of HIV and its medicalisation do not seem to have reduced, or removed, HIV related stigma, just relegated it to a minor issue of less importance. Interestingly, Varas-Diaz et al. (2005) note 'because of the expected increase in HIV cases by the year 2020, the stigma surrounding it is likely to intensify' (Varas-Diaz et al., 2005, p. 169). HIV related stigma is often experienced within employment, housing, health services and indeed from social contexts such as from family and friends (Herek et al. 2002). Stigma frames many aspects of the HIV epidemic, perhaps most obviously in the lives of those people living with the virus but also, to some extent, wider populations. HIV related stigma leads to delays in HIV testing in many countries (see, for example, Chesney and Smith, 1999; Myers et al., 1993; Stall et al., 1996).

Conclusion

This chapter has outlined some of the 'everyday problems' of living with HIV in the UK in the twenty-first century (Green and Smith, 2004). It presents the 'aftermath' of effective and transformative medical developments and a corresponding reduction in HIV morbidity and mortality. Yet it also traces the persistence and growth of other transitions within HIV management: the relegation of the psychosocial in relation to the primacy of the medical and public health. This 'welcome' but sometimes problematic shift means new resonances with wider fields of literature: an engagement with issues of chronic illness rather than palliative care, or end of life studies. Yet despite the apparent 'normalisation' of HIV in the West (DeCock and Johnson, 1998) the exceptionalism of HIV is still apparent. Effective treatment for HIV may indeed have normalised the medical care and management of infection, yet for many people living with HIV there are on-going and even newly developing psychosocial challenges.

The brief history of HIV includes its transformation in the West from terminal disease to chronic manageable condition and from death sentence to life sentence (Flowers et al., 2001, p. 669). A diversification of illness trajectories follows in which mortality and morbidity are shaped according to both time period and current access to wealth and health care. This chapter has shown that for very different people all living with HIV in the UK now, these histories have palpable contemporary consequences; their lives are haunted by the spirits of HIV both past and future. Irrespective of demographic or cultural background, there is a consistent sense of the contingent meaning of HIV diagnosis. This uncertainty, often in relation to ideas of self or identity, represents the particular ontological burden of living with HIV. This uncertainty contrasts sharply with the immutable medical certainty of the process of diagnosis, the tangible veracity and regularity of the hard biomedical truth of HIV and its requirements of daily doses of toxic chemicals (ART).

Moreover, through this particular lens, processes of HIV 'normalisation' (DeCock and Johnson, 1998) seem to have been confounded with HIV medicalisation and the resulting minimisation of psychosocial understandings of HIV. The latter, so salient in earlier eras in which effective treatment for HIV were not available, are now often overshadowed or dismissed as less important than medical health outcome measures.

References

Blanch J., Rousaud, A., Martínez, E., De Lazzari, E., Peri, J., Milinkovic, A., Perez-Cuevas, J., Blanco, J., Gatell, J. (2002) 'Impact of lipodystrophy on the quality of life of HIV-1-infected patients', *Journal of Acquired Immune Deficiency Syndromes*, 31, 4, 404–7.

Brashers, D., Neidig, N., Cardillo, N., Dobbs, L., Russell, J. A. and Haas, S. M. (1999) '"In an important way, I did die": uncertainty and revival in persons living with HIV or AIDS', *AIDS Care*, 11, 201–9.

Chesney, M. A. and Smith, A. W. (1999) 'Critical delays in HIV testing and care: the potential role of stigma', *American Behavioural Scientist*, 42, 1162–74.

Ciesla, J. and Roberts, J. (2001) 'Meta-analysis of the relationship between HIV Infection and risk for depressive disorders', *American Journal of Psychiatry*, 158, 725–30.

Collins, E., Wagner, C. and Walmsley, M. (2000) 'Psychosocial impact of the lipidystrophy syndrome in HIV infection', *AIDS Reader*, 10, 9, 546–51.

DeCock, K. and Johnson, A. (1998) 'From exceptionalism to normalisation: a reappraisal of attitudes and practice around HIV testing', *British Medical Journal*, 316, 290–3.

Ezzy, D. (2000), 'Illness narratives: time, hope and HIV', *Social Science and Medicine*, 50, 605–17.

Flowers, P., Duncan, B. and Knussen, C. (2001) 'Re-appraising HIV testing amongst Scottish gay men: the impact of new treatments', *Journal of Health Psychology*, 6, 665–79.

Garcia, F., De Lazzari, E., Plana, M., Castro, P., Mestre, G. and Nomdedeu, M. (2004) 'Long-term CD4+ T-cell response to highly active antiretroviral therapy according to baseline CD4+ T-cell count', *Journal of Acquired Immune Deficiency Syndrome*, 36, 702–13.

Green, G. and Smith, R. (2004) 'The psychosocial and health care needs of HIV positive people in the UK: a review', *HIV Medicine*, 5, 5–46.

Gulick, R. M., Meibohm, A., Havlir, D., Eron, J. J., Mosley, A. and Chodakewitz, J. A. (2003) 'Six-year follow-up of HIV-1-infected adults in a clinical trial of antiretroviral therapy with indinavir, zidovudine, and lamivudine', *AIDS*, 17, 2345–9.

Herek, G., Capitano J. P. and Widaman, K. F. (2002). 'HIV-Related Stigma and Knowledge in the United States: Prevalence and Trends, 1991–1999', *American Journal of Public Health*, 92, 371–7.

Kalichman, S. and Sikkema, K. (1994) 'Psychological sequelae of HIV-infection and AIDS – review of empirical-findings', *Clinical Psychology Review*, 14, 7, 611–32.

Katz, I. and Wright, A. (2008) 'Circumcision — a surgical strategy for HIV prevention in Africa', *New England Journal of Medicine*, 359, 2412–15.

Kaufmann, G. R., Perrin, L., Pantaleo, G., Opravil, M., Furrer, H. and Telenti, A., (2003) 'CD4 T-lymphocyte recovery in individuals with advanced HIV-1 infection receiving potent antiretroviral therapy for 4 years: the Swiss HIV Cohort Study', *Archives of Internal Medicine*, 163, 2187–95.

Myers, T., Orr, K. W., Locker, D. and Jackson, E. A. (1993) 'Factors affecting gay and bisexual men's decisions and intentions to seek HIV testing', *American Journal of Public Health*, 83,701–4.

Pierret, J. (2001) 'Interviews and biographical time: the case of longterm HIV nonprogressors', *Sociology of Health & Illness*, 23, 159–79.

Roth, N. and Nelson, M. (1994) 'HIV diagnosis rituals and HIV identity narratives', *AIDS Care*, 9, 161–80.

Scambler, G. (1998) 'Stigma and disease: changing paradigms', *Lancet*, 352, 1054–5.

Siegel, K. and Lekas, H. (2002) 'AIDS as a chronic illness: psychosocial implications', *AIDS*, 16, S69–S76.

Smith, J. A., Flowers, P. and Larkin, M. (2009) *Interpretative Phenomenological Analysis: Method and Research* (London: Sage).

Stall, R., Hoff, C., Coates, T. J., Paul, J., Phillips, K., Ekstrand, M., Kegeles, S., Catania, J., Daigle, D., Diaz, R. (1996) 'Decisions to get HIV tested and to accept antiretroviral therapies among gay/bisexual men: implications for secondary prevention efforts', *Journal of Acquired Immune Deficiency Syndromes and Human Retrovirology*, 11, 151–60.

Tewksbury, R. and McGaughey, D. (1998) 'Identities and identity transformations among persons with HIV disease', *International Journal of Sexuality and Gender Studies*, 3, 213–32.

Treichler, P. (1987) 'AIDS, homophobia and biomedical discourse: an epidemic of signification', *Cultural Studies*, 1, 263–305.

Varas-Díaz, N., Serrano-García, I. and Toro-Alfonso, J. (2005) 'AIDS-related stigma and social interaction: Puerto Ricans living with HIV/AIDS', *Qualitative Health Research*, 15, 2, 169–87.

7

Antiretroviral Treatment and HIV Prevention: Perspectives from Qualitative Research with Gay Men with HIV in the UK

Mark Davis

Introduction

> the reason that I'm confused at the moment is because of a remark made to me by [my doctor] when I actually raised my sexual behaviour as an issue during the clinical session .... He said that I was more, I had more chance of passing on hepatitis B than I did of passing on HIV given the low detectable, the undetectable level of my viral load .... I walk about with those words reverberating in my head, not knowing whether I can believe them or not .... I've no idea because my medical knowledge isn't developed enough to know.
>
> (Alasdair: 1)[1]

This is an extract from an interview regarding the implications of antiretroviral treatment (ART) for the risk of transmission in sexual intercourse. It comes from research I will consider in later parts of the chapter. The quotation concerns the idea that undetectable viral load, one of the desired effects of ART, implies that the risk of HIV transmission is reduced. As such, it reflects a narrative that recognises the advent of ART as a biotechnological watershed in the epidemic with implications for knowledge concerning the action of HIV in bodies, its status as a biological entity and for social responses to the epidemic. Alasdair's expression of confusion raises the themes I want to address. He makes a division between his own and medical expertise, suggesting the challenge of engaging with the knowledge and effects pertaining to ART and HIV prevention. However, the advice from the medical expert is represented as the source of confusion, so we are led to the view that technical considerations and expertise are not the only issues here. Further, 'not knowing whether I can believe them or not' expresses awareness of the potentially controversial implications of the medical expert's perspective. Alasdair's account acknowledges that reduced risk of HIV transmission has implications for sexual relations. But, it also underlines that the technical appraisal of the relative risk of HIV and hepatitis B transmission is not, in and of itself, an answer to the question of how to act. In this way, the technical aspects of the knowledge systems of ART and implications for the risk of HIV transmission articulate with, but are distinct from, the ethical implications of such knowledge for sexual relations.

Such questions of ethical social action can be considered in light of what Nikolas Rose has termed 'informational biocitizenship' (2007: 135). Rose used this term to draw attention to the relational and collective practices produced through interests in, and the circulation of, biotechnological knowledge and effects. Examples noted by Rose include HIV treatment advocacy movements (2007). Informational biocitizenship connects biotechnology with the Foucauldian concept of technologies of self. In this view, biotechnologies, among other features of contemporary society, assist 'individuals to effect by their own means or with the help of others a certain number of operations on their own bodies and souls, thoughts conduct and way of being' (Foucault, 1988: 18). Rose however draws attention to the struggles, debates and controversies related to biotechnological knowledge and effects. The example provided by Alasdair is salient. It implies that knowledge regarding the relative risk of HIV and hepatitis B, and the articulation of these with HIV prevention, create ethical dilemmas. Alasdair's question to himself, 'not knowing whether I can believe them or not', is a form of self-subjection that heavily underlines how ethical concerns embrace but exceed technical information. Although the knowledge produced by biotechnology is not ostensibly a guide to action, the circulation of such knowledge serves to sharpen the ethical questions for the patient/citizen. Accordingly, this chapter considers the merit of the informational biocitizenship perspective in an analysis of narratives regarding living with ART and implications for preventing HIV transmission in sexual practice.

The interviews I will draw on here were conducted in London between 1999 and 2000 with gay men with HIV. Some of these interviews were undertaken for SHARP, a quantitative and qualitative research project addressing the impact of ART on sexual behaviour (Stephenson et al., 2003). Repeat interviews with the same participants were conducted for my doctoral studies at the Institute of Education, University of London[1].

The research is a useful case study for this volume. Gay men remain one of the groups in the UK most affected by HIV. By end 2007, it was reported that there were 77,400 people living with HIV in the UK (Health Protection Agency, 2008). Of these, 30,800 were gay and other homosexually active men, 16,900 were African born women and 8,950 were African born men. These numbers regarding African born people mirror the higher impact of the HIV epidemic on women in other parts of the world. Of the gay and other homosexually active men newly diagnosed in 2007, an estimated 82% acquired their infection in the UK. By contrast, it is reported that 77% of newly diagnosed heterosexual men and women acquired their infection outside the UK. SHARP was conducted soon after the introduction of ART in the mid- to late-1990s in the UK and also after reports of escalation in reported unsafe sex among gay men in London and in other cities around the globe (Elford, 2006). SHARP was designed to address the notion that the introduction of ART was contributing to the escalation in reported sexual risk behaviour. At that time it was hypothesised that optimistic beliefs regarding the effects of ART on the risk of HIV transmission were leading gay men to give up condoms for anal sex. A central concept in this research was 'treatment optimism', derived from health psychology, and in particular, the Health Belief Model (HBM). Among its perspectives, the HBM assumes that fear motivates individuals to cease dangerous, and adopt protective, behaviours. Treatment optimism is based on this idea. It was postulated that as the dangers of HIV infection subsided due to ART and in accord with the HBM, sexual intercourse without condoms would increase. Since SHARP, research from different parts of the world has shown that treatment optimism does not explain changes in condom use particularly well. For example, there does appear to be an association between endorsing treatment optimism and self-reported sex without condoms, but as Jonathan Elford has pointed out, treatment optimism may be an *ex post facto* rationalisation that reduces anxiety regarding risky sex (Elford, 2006). The quantitative analysis from SHARP showed that, compared with those not on treatment, those on treatment were less likely to report unsafe sex (Stephenson et al., 2003). A review of research in developing countries found that ART was associated with a *reduction* in sexual behaviours that would transmit HIV, although the authors based their findings on the three research articles that met their inclusion criteria, all of which derived from Africa (Kennedy et al., 2007). It is also plain that treatment optimism, derived as it is from notions of fear avoidance, does not help explain how people who already know they have HIV infection engage with the impact of ART in HIV prevention. In addition, the SHARP interviews suggested that the treatment optimism thesis was crude (Davis et al., 2002). The interviewees engaged with the implications of ART in ways that were not understandable in light of treatment optimism. As Alasdair's example shows, engagements are informed by a complex of changing technical knowledge, the social relations of biotechnological expertise and ethical dilemmas wrought at the intersection of medical and public health discourses.

This chapter takes up Alasdair's 'confusion' and related examples to explore bioinformational ethics regarding ART and HIV prevention. This is an analytical project that necessarily considers medical technologies and the expert knowledge systems that bring their effects into being, public health engagements with these systems in relation to the risk of HIV transmission and the ethical questions that arise. By drawing on the SHARP interviews, in the sections to follow I will argue that

- the impact of ART on HIV prevention is informed by a narrative of medically determined watershed, but also that, alternative stories of living with ART question the singular, normalising properties of the ART story;
- the ART narrative has the dual effect of forcing those with HIV infection living in developed countries onto their personal resources while encouraging public and policy views that HIV is a manageable infection and thus normalised. In these circumstances, people determine methods of living with ART that comprise personalised, but hidden, 'technologies of hope' that also provide a pattern for the informational ethics of ART and HIV prevention; and
- because technical information regarding the impact of ART on HIV prevention does not in and of itself address questions of social action, people with HIV are required to translate the effects of ART for the risk of transmission in sexual relations. In this situation, the personalising, hidden implications of ART for the person with HIV are brought into connection with the ethical implications for sexual relating. It also appears that the production and dissemination of technical knowledge in the ART clinic is ambiguous, deepening the challenges of informational biocitizenship.

Narrative alterities

It is often taken as axiomatic that ART has transformed the HIV epidemic. According to this understanding, ART is a medical breakthrough (often dated to the mid-1990s) that has altered the course of the epidemic and also the lives of the individuals affected by it. It is of course not my interest to dispute the effects of ART on the health of those who can get access to it. But I want to investigate how this watershed assumption is invested in a particular ordering of the relationships between HIV treatment, prevention and ethical citizenship. While ART has had dramatic effects for many of those who can have access to it, the watershed narrative is not universal. For example, Corinne Squire has shown how responses to the epidemic in South Africa in the post-ART era reveal a mixture of engagements with the prospect of being able to control HIV infection through ART in situations where access to it is uneven, uncertain or absent; struggles to speak out about living with HIV and community-based campaigns advocating for treatment access where government figures have dismissed them as instruments of neo-colonialism (2007). I want to take this instructive complexity into an analysis of the stories of gay men with HIV living in London. As we will see, it is possible to trace the effects of the ART watershed narrative into the treatment/prevention relationship and the 'personalising' aspects of ART. In addition, I want to show how the watershed narrative can be contrasted with other possible and necessary narratives of transition into (and in) the post-ART period. These other stories reveal the normalising power of the ART watershed narrative and related implications for informational biocitizenship.

The ART watershed narrative is important to the relationship between HIV treatment and prevention and, in particular, the concept of treatment optimism. Before ART, the lack of a solution for HIV was regarded as a crisis for those affected by HIV, but also for medicine because it was unable to meet its promise of conquering disease. This lack gave HIV prevention its value and urgency, but also tied it closely to the failure and success of medicine in relation to HIV. In the post-ART period, HIV prevention necessarily requires a new justification that takes account of effective treatment. The concept of treatment optimism, and through it the HBM, supplies such justification. It can be argued that the HBM itself arose because of questions to do with biotechnologies and preventative medicine. As Irwin Rosenstock pointed out years ago, the HBM was developed to address what was seen as the failure on the part of some people to take up polio vaccination (1974). The concept of treatment optimism, drawing as it does on the HBM, makes the link between prevention and treatment through a focus on sexual practice and ART. For people living in developed countries, and to some extent in developing countries, there has been copious research regarding perceptions of the effects of ART on the risk of transmission and sexual practice (Elford, 2006). We could also argue that treatment optimism research addresses the excess of hope for a biotechnological solution to the epidemic. Foucault famously noted how end of plague festivals, with all their masking and unmasking of identities and unruly mixing of bodies, served as a counterpoint to the governance necessary to deal with plague (1982: 197). Quite literally, the 'optimism' in treatment optimism marks the excess of hope implied in ART. But research regarding treatment optimism also represents an attempt to solve what is seen as the problem of end-of-plague unruliness. This anxiety is also expressed in other contexts, where ART is not readily available. For example, the expansion of ART provision in developing countries is often questioned on the basis of speculations – with no current empirical basis – that it will lead to increased risky behaviours (Kennedy et al., 2007).

One other important aspect of the ART watershed narrative, as it is expressed in developed country contexts, is to deepen the personalisation of HIV infection while, at the same time, extending the notion that HIV is a manageable, 'less crisis', disease. As many others have noted, the AIDS crisis story has proved hard to sustain, or even undesirable, in developed country contexts with access to ART (Race, 2001; Rofes, 1998). Simon Watney has noted: 'Most people no longer speak of AIDS as a crisis. It has become part of the general social and mental furniture of our times' (2000: 260). International NGOs have found it difficult to sustain the sense of crisis that existed in the 1980s. Policy analysts have recognised the 'normalisation' of HIV in health care around the globe (Rosenbrock et al., 2000). Others have argued on medical grounds, and in particular because of the advent of ART, for the active normalisation of aspects of HIV care such as antibody testing (De Cock and Johnson, 1998). At the same time and adopting the frame of medicalisation, researchers have argued that using HIV-related technologies, such as ART, strengthens the importance of engagements with clinical expertise and also deepens the individualising aspects of living with HIV. As Paul Flowers has noted, such individualising takes the form of increased emphasis on personal responsibility in matters of health care and the erosion of community-based social support for people with HIV (Flowers, 2001; Flowers et al., 2001). Indeed, during the late 1990s and early 2000s in the UK, voluntary sector community-support services, such as Body Positive in London, ceased to function or were absorbed into HIV agencies. Flowers has also noted that the individualisation of living with HIV in the UK is set against public complacency with regard to the HIV epidemic itself. As an interviewee in the SHARP research put it:

> how am I going to cope with life not being under a death sentence? What do I do now? Because, you know, the other thing is, you can't

> quite believe that's where you are, because we are not there yet, that's the thing ... so when you hear the friggin' Daily Mail say, you know: 'AIDS is now a manageable condition like diabetes'. You think: 'Yes, well, no, actually, no'. Treatments fail. People have problems. People have to come off treatments. Things go wrong. What do you do then?
>
> (Michael: 2)

This quotation suggests the separation between public and personal aspects of the post-ART experience. In the news, the HIV epidemic is tucked inside 'manageable disease'. Lived experience however, appears more provisional.

In addition, the ART watershed is one possible narrative among several. As interviews from the SHARP research revealed, other narrative forms include a traditional form of 'body blow', a more metaphysical sense of prophecy and a risk-oriented exchange of liminalities. These different stories suggest the necessary engagement with, or even invention of, informational ethics for the situation of changing options regarding the treatment of HIV infection. Several SHARP interviewees made reference to ART watershed narrative, for example,

> I had the HIV test and it came back positive and I just wasn't expecting it at all, and so I didn't drink, but I smoked more and more and more, thinking I'd be dead in two years ... in 1991 it was HIV equals AIDS equals death.
>
> (Michael: 2)

In this example, Michael referred to a period of the HIV epidemic when there was no effective treatment: 'it was AZT, there was no other hope and that wasn't a hope you know. Everyone I knew on AZT was dying' (Michael: 2). However and in contrast with straightforward turnaround narrative, it was also possible to exceed the poor life expectations of that period: 'when I was diagnosed I was given five years and I superseded that by one year. I'm overdue death by one year' (Michael: 2). This quotation and others like it positioned the authors as the beneficiaries of superseded predictions or as incredulous observers of their own survival. Importantly, these experiences were not always attached to the advent of ART, as, like Michael, some interviewees made reference to situations where they had already exceeded prognoses when they began ART. There was also a suggestion that such changes referred to the reputation of HIV treatments such as AZT. AZT was tried as a treatment for HIV in the late 1980s and early 1990s without success. In combination with other ARTs however, AZT has had some benefits. So it can also be argued that ART watershed narrative implies a reversal in the reputation of treatment technology per se. Further support for narrative alterity in the post-ART period can be found in accounts of people living with HIV in South Africa. As Squire has pointed out in the South Africa context, improved life prospects are not only linked with ART. Campaigns combating HIV stigma flowing into improved access to prophylaxis for opportunistic infections, prevention of mother-to-child transmission (PMTCT), and the adoption of safer sex have had putative effects in HIV morbidity (2007). In addition, the effects of these programmes have synergies with, and extend the effects of, ART.

In contrast with turnaround, Kevin provided an account where he was diagnosed with HIV infection after ART became available and at a time when he needed it immediately. Kevin spoke of realising that he 'actually might die' (1) but that through treatment he was able to return to work. In this account, the experience of illness and diagnosis is positioned after the ART watershed. A relatively sudden and life-threatening illness was depicted as the 'body blow' (2) that precipitated diagnosis and therefore altered the life-course. This kind of account therefore deploys a traditional illness narrative (Hyden, 1997). Another possible story of living in post-ART was a kind of prophecy of infection.

> I remember being at school and our science teacher said we were discussing the, you know, HIV had just come out, and he said at least one person in this classroom will be HIV positive, you know it's inevitable
>
> (Edgar: 2)

This account turned the science of prediction into a sense of the inevitable, as if risk calculations revealed individual fate. This depiction of experience was not turnaround or biographical disruption as such. For example, according to Edgar it was 'really difficult to pinpoint any major change in my life' (2). Prophecy makes HIV infection seem to be part of the order of nature and history, or outside of reflexivity. Central here is the idea that sexual activity in a high HIV prevalence sexual community increases the risk of HIV transmission to the point that it is not avoidable. Another accounting strategy involved moving from one liminal state to another.

> I knew what I had done, I sort of suspected I probably was HIV positive, but whilst I was, I felt well I don't see the need to have a test, which I don't now agree with really, but then thinking about it, at the time there was, treatment was sort of very much in its infancy. So maybe I was right, I don't know
>
> (Robert: 2)

Robert gave an impression that he diagnosed himself and delayed testing until he was confident with ART. Robert's account traces out a strategy for dealing with HIV that moves from living with the possibility of HIV infection to living with the possibility of treatment.

Self-treating subjectivity

Narrative alterity counterpoints the idea of a universal, medicalised post-ART experience. These stories also form a point of contrast with the developing world context where access to ART is uneven and uncertain. In this context, people live with ART in highly politicised ways, locally, nationally and internationally. Medical HIV technologies of diagnosis, treatment and care are often necessarily and effectively dispersed beyond the clinic to community-based organisations and families (Abdullah and Squire, this volume; Colvin and Robins, 2009; Farmer, 1999). For those with HIV in developed countries (who can get access to ART), personalised engagements with medical technologies combined with public normalisation imply that people with HIV are forced onto their own resources. As is well documented in the literature, the uncertainties of ART can be a considerable challenge both for patients (Davis et al., 2006) and prescribers (Rosengarten et al., 2004). SHARP interviewees suggested that in such circumstances caring for the self necessitated finding methods for cultivating and sustaining mind, body and soul to optimise the 'positive uncertainties' of ART. These ways of living with ART had ethical resonances in the Foucauldian sense of technologies of the self and therefore informational biocitizenship (1988).

The self-care methods offered by the interviewees comprised planning, positioning, conserving, settling and normalising. The methods reveal how, in various ways or with various emphases, the self with HIV 'invests' in, or furthers an engagement with ART that serves to draw attention to or optimise its positive effects. As such, the methods are open-ended: they are ongoing and have no closure. One approach was to develop a planned approach to self-care.

> then I had my game plan for the future, which was look after myself, I mean this probably means a bit more, is actually take bad use of bad word, positive steps to look after myself as opposed to let my whim look after myself. This is going to the gym
>
> (Stephen: 2)

Such self-care could also be turned to caring for and improving the interior, psychological self.

> the way to prevent the onset of AIDS was about living a healthy lifestyle in every way ... cut out a lot of the toxins ... working on lots of mental issues all of my past and clearing all of the garbage out
>
> (Michael: 2)

This account suggests an aesthetic value of purity of body and mind. This was a kind of placing oneself in the best possible position to deal with HIV infection and to optimise ART. Another method was collecting the self, for example, 'I've learned to be a great conservator' (Kevin: 2). Relevant techniques included distractions, reinforcing 'easily achievable targets', striving for 'psychic balance', being aware of negative thoughts and rethinking social relationships (Kevin: 2). Self-care was informed by the idea that HIV disease had become a 'potential' rather than an actuality.

> I think the whole question of HIV treatment and what helps HIV positive patients is in such a state of flux now because instead of being basket cases they've all become people carrying the potential to be a basket case but who can go straight back into life. And I don't know of any other illness where we have any kind of parallel learning that we could transfer over about how people are meant to cope with that. And so I think we're all on new territory, and it's pretty tough territory.
>
> (Kevin: 2)

This account underlined the precarious and personal quality of living with ART that led into a kind of vigilant, resigned, conservation of self. A harmonising survival method was also reflected in accounts of living with ART. Stephen spoke of taking treatment as a 'settlement period where I actually felt comfortable and I realised that I'd got all this sorted out because I wasn't getting ill' (2). Stephen spoke of wanting 'a settled life' (2). There was some ambiguity to this use of 'settlement' where it could mean that a future was stable but also that it was laid out in a certain way.

Andrew used similar words, saying that he was 'more centred', 'content' and 'calmer' (2). Yet another self-care method was normalisation. It was typified by 'I try to let things wash over me' (Robert: 2) or 'I don't let it get on top of me, deal with it now and then, it's fine' (Andrew: 2) and 'I think I've grown into it ... I'd say I've got used to it' (Andrew: 2). Similarly, regarding AIDS as extraordinary was not relevant:

> Robert: ... and I'm sort of more disciplined about doing exercise. But, you know, you should be anyway really, so I feel good after I've done exercise.
>
> MD: But have you instituted these practices because of HIV or ...
>
> Robert: Yeah, initially it was because of HIV I think, but it's sort of become a routine if you like ... sort of a way of life really. So I'm not sort of conscious, I'm not thinking oh I must go to the swimming pool to exercise because of my HIV, you know, I'm not really very conscious of it. And people say the drugs are a constant reminder, I don't think so. I mean I take vitamins every morning, you know, and you don't think about it do you, what you're taking and why ...
>
> (2)

In this strategy, the ART experience is depicted as non-exceptional. Self-care was figured as routine. In this orientation to living with HIV, a normative healthy self is a reference point for self-care activity. And this normal self is achieved by bracketing out HIV. Robert's example of normalisation turns us back to the hidden, personalised forms of self-care that are necessary for ART. Normalisation also refers to policy and cultural formations of HIV as unexceptional. Via these various 'technologies of hope', we could argue that, for some in the developed country context at least, the labour of ART is turned to making AIDS invisible. Another relevant perspective here is that living with HIV carries social stigma, as has been recognised since the beginning of the epidemic in developed and developing country contexts (Herdt, 2001). 'Invisibility' is thus also required, or even desirable, to manage stigma and prejudice. The labour of taking ART is thus ambiguously onerous and beneficial, but nevertheless works to deepen hidden, personalised self-care.

These observations regarding invisible and individualised HIV treatment connect with the notion of loss of community interest in relation to HIV in developed country contexts. It is possible to argue that treatment advocacy, at least in developed countries, has given way to a focus on treatment compliance, side effects and other aspects of the management of ART (Green and Smith, 2004). In relation to HIV prevention, some have argued that collective action has been displaced by individualised action in gay communities (Adam, 2005; Sheon and Crosby, 2004), making HIV prevention less visible. These articulations of biotechnology and (in)visibility are relevant in situations where access to HIV treatment is uneven or uncertain, but take a different form. For example, many have acknowledged that despite efforts to develop HIV treatment and prevention in parallel, improved ART provision is being matched by 'faltering' prevention initiatives, whose technologies are harder to define, evidence, deliver and scale up (Global HIV Prevention Working Group, 2007). HIV prevention is therefore 'disappearing' in its earlier forms, and in its newer incarnations, adopting biomedical processes of founding itself on evidence bases, scaling up from pilots and operating with firm protocols, ongoing evaluation and strict targets. In relation to these examples, we could argue therefore that there is a general pattern of (in)visible, disappearing or biotechnologised HIV prevention, articulated alongside biotechnological innovation.

ART, sex and clinical expertise

While living with ART can be said to comprise personalised, invisibilised technologies of hope, HIV prevention requires social actors to discuss HIV with their sexual partners, or at least, consider it as part of the negotiation of sex. Therefore, people using ART have to translate the personalising implications of ART for the situation of sexual relations. As we will see, the ART watershed narrative makes an appearance here as an important way of addressing the informational ethics that arise at the intersection of ART and HIV prevention. Because it is the source of technical knowledge, the clinic is also important. As I have discussed, technical knowledge regarding the impact of ART on the risk of HIV transmission does not necessarily resolve HIV prevention concerns, although it does sharpen ethical considerations. But in addition, the ethical challenge for sexual citizenship is amplified because there is also contest over technical knowledge regarding ART and HIV prevention, in some situations attributed to clinical expertise, as Alasdair's extract demonstrates. These aspects of technical knowledge reflect what Flowers (2001: 63) has called the 'fracturing' of, and Rosengarten et al. (2001: 4) have called 'individually tailored' approaches to, HIV prevention in the post-ART situation. As with living with ART, people with HIV turn back onto themselves in matters of ART, HIV prevention and sexual relations, but they also draw on dialogues with clinical expertise. Such collaboration is said to be a desirable feature of HIV treatment in general (Persson et al., 2003; Rosengarten et al., 2004). What is distinctive here is how clinical expertise is entered into questions of citizenship regarding ART and sexual practice.

Two contrasting accounts serve to draw attention to the informational ethics implied by ART and HIV prevention. These accounts refer to the risk of HIV transmission to a sexual partner who also has HIV infection, known as reinfection. There is considerable debate with regard to the health implications of re-infection, reflected in research (Porco et al., 2004) and policy (Bernard, 2008). In the following extract, the interviewee makes reference to a decision regarding condom use with another man with HIV.

> Robert: As regards the HIV, I suppose really we should have got our doctors to put their heads together and find out if we had the same strain of the virus, but I was strongly inclined to feel that we did have.
>
> MD: How come?
>
> Robert: I think we were sort of infected at about the same time. I don't know, it's a silly assumption really isn't it? You know, it wasn't sort of based on anything, sort of scientific fact. But you know I spoke to my doctor here about it: 'What do you think about us having unprotected sex?' And he said: 'Well I would go ahead. I really wouldn't worry about it.'
>
> (1)

This account combines advice from a physician with a notion that the interviewee's virus and that of his partner were 'the same' in terms of both genotype ('strain') and a temporal ordering of the epidemic ('time'). These judgements of viral equivalence reveal an assumption of one epidemic over linear time, implying the ART watershed narrative. Equivalence relies on an ordering of bodies in epidemic time, in particular, in terms of the advent of ART. Preventing HIV becomes a matter of determining sameness and difference when considering HIV prevention in relation to someone else with HIV infection. In this account, however, sex without condoms with another man with HIV was seen as a source of concern.

> Well, when we both found out we were positive, we used condoms at first and then he kept saying: 'You don't have to use condoms', and

> I said: 'I can reinfect you and you can reinfect me', I said, 'I don't think it's a good idea'. But we did actually. We did about three or four times, we did have unprotected sex ... I thought: 'Well, no, I'm just not sure, I can't afford to catch really, anything, or make things, matters worse.'
>
> (Philip: 1)

The contrast between these accounts suggests the articulation of different preferences for managing HIV prevention that resemble the personalised technologies of hope already discussed. These examples also draw attention to the relational aspects of HIV prevention, including both the sexual partnership and engagement with medical experts. They stress how managing the risk of reinfection implies social negotiation of expert knowledge, shaded personal preferences and the articulation of these with a desire to achieve a sense of security in sexual practice.

Another pair of contrasting examples serve to underline how technical knowledge is itself open to contestation. They suggest that the provision of advice regarding the impact of ART on HIV prevention may not be uniform. They also suggest that ART creates a situation of different bodies with different biomedical characteristics and therefore different implications for risk of HIV transmission in sex. Colin had this to say with regard to ART and HIV transmission.

> I was part of the control group because I didn't have gonorrhoea (laughs) and he [researcher] came back and said we can't find any virus in your semen or sperm. I was quite shocked actually by that but I have read things in the papers and magazines over the years of being just left in the spleen and the tonsils. So why not just have one's spleen and tonsils out and be done with it!
>
> (Colin: 1)

In the next account, the interviewee also refers to being provided with advice. In this instance however, the interviewee suggests that treatment does not necessarily reduce infectiousness.

> from speaking to [my doctor] and from my own reading around the subject it seems that a low viral load in your blood system is no guarantee that there's no HIV in your semen or that there's a similarly low reading of HIV there. And my understanding also is that even if the drugs penetrate your blood stream so as to suppress HIV there that it can be in all sorts of other places, like your brain and

> lymphatic system. So I don't assume that 'cause I've got a low viral load that I can screw people without risking them I don't think.
>
> (Kevin: 1)

One common social science understanding of engagements with knowledge systems, such as those that support ART, is that individuals vary in their capacity to access, recall and apply information. As this chapter has argued, technical knowledge in and of itself does not address how to act. The examples of Robert, Philip, Colin and Kevin underline how the ethical questions for sexual relating produced by ART knowledge and effects require reference to clinical expertise articulated with the idiosyncratic aspects of ART. Further, because expertise is shown to vary, these considerations are necessarily open to revision. These examples underline how ART and its implications for HIV prevention imply informational biocitizenship, with pronounced relational dimensions involving clinical encounters and sexual relations.

Conclusion

This chapter took Alasdair's 'confusion' to imply that the impact of ART in HIV prevention embraces, but exceeds, biotechnical considerations. I used the notion of informational biocitizenship to help conceptualise this field of action. The example of treatment optimism, which offers limited forms of explanation even by its own criteria, has been shown to express the excess of hope for a biotechnological approach to the HIV epidemic and through it, anxiety and consternation with regard to the challenge of governing HIV transmission in the post-ART era. I traced informational ethics into the other stories of living with ART and into the personalised 'technologies of hope' that sustain ways of living with ART. I also considered the translation work undertaken by people using ART to do with acknowledging and supporting the effects of ART on HIV in individual bodies and reflecting on the complexities and ambiguities of the implications of such knowledge for the risk of HIV transmission in their sexual relations.

As I have argued, and in accord with other case studies in this volume, understanding the links between HIV treatment and prevention requires that we re-examine prevailing assumptions and methods of analysis. For example, an orthodox approach to the confusion expressed by Alasdair would be to provide him with further, better, more up-to-date information, perhaps fixed in the form of a pamphlet or online, interactive resource. Some might even argue for the chastisement of his clinical adviser for apparently providing such bald information regarding undetectable viral load, and perhaps, elaborate professional education for clinicians with regard to such matters. Some might even take the position that, because these technical and ethical concerns are so complex, such discussions should never happen lest the clinic be the source of a kind of iatrogenic HIV epidemic. As this case study has shown, such approaches are not likely to resolve such concerns. The dissemination of technical information regarding ART and its implications for HIV prevention is always-already, and inescapably, ethical. More, not less, conversation is called for regarding the positioning of people with HIV, their sexual partners, clinicians and others, in this field of HIV-related informational biocitizenship. Such negotiations of citizenship have found expression in, for example, community-accountable models of ART adherence support in the Western Cape in South Africa (Squire, 2007). Other chapters in this volume also make reference to the need to address questions of citizenship in HIV prevention (see Cathy Campbell and Lindy Wilbraham, this volume). Such examples and the analysis presented here reveal that there is much to be gained from taking informational biocitizenship as a starting point in discourse regarding the connections between ART and prevention. In particular, we can now understand that 'confusion' is not simply produced by a lack of information, a failure of expertise, overwhelming biotechnological complexity, or a problem in the clinical encounter. Confusion as such is an invitation to discourse regarding the 'extra-technical' dimensions of ethical self-governance produced at the intersection of HIV treatment and prevention technologies.

Acknowledgements

I would like to thank my colleagues from the SHARP Project (Sexual risk behaviour and relation to antiretroviral therapy in HIV positive gay men project, UK Medical Research Council, Grant: G98116 43): Judith Stephenson (Principal Investigator), John Imrie (Principal Investigator), Graham Hart (Investigator), Oliver Davidson (Investigator), Ian Williams (Investigator). I am also very grateful for the interviewees who offered their support for SHARP and my doctoral research.

References

Adam, B. (2005) 'Constructing the neoliberal sexual actor: responsibility and care of the self in the discourse of barebackers', *Culture, Health and Sexuality*, 7, 4, 333–46.

Bernard, E. (2008) 'Swiss experts say individuals with undetectable viral load and no STI cannot transmit HIV during sex', *Aidsmap News*, www.aidsmap.com, 31 January 2008.

Colvin, C. and Robins, S. (2009) 'Social movements and HIV-AIDS in South Africa', in P. Rohleder, L. Swartz, S. Kalichman and L. Simbayi (eds) *HIV/AIDS in South Africa 25 years on: psychosocial perspectives* (New York: Springer).

Davis, M., Frankis, J. and Flowers, P. (2006) 'Uncertainty and technological horizon in qualitative interviews about HIV treatment', *Health: An Interdisciplinary Journal for the Social Study of Health, Illness and Medicine*, 10, 3, 323–44.

Davis, M., Hart, G., Imrie, J., Davidson, O., Williams, I. and Stephenson, J. (2002) '"HIV is HIV to me": meanings of treatments, viral load and reinfection among gay men with HIV', *Health, Risk and Society*, 4, 1, 31–43.

De Cock, K. and Johnson, A. (1998) 'From exceptionalism to normalisation: a reappraisal of attitudes and practice around HIV testing', *British Medical Journal*, 316, 290–3.

Elford, J. (2006) 'Changing patterns of sexual behaviour in the era of highly active antiretroviral therapy', *Current Opinion in Infectious Diseases*, 19, 26–32.

Farmer, P. (1999) *Infections and inequalities* (Berkeley, CA: University of California Press).

Flowers, P. (2001) 'Gay men and HIV/AIDS risk management', *Health*, 5, 50–75.

Flowers, P., Knussen, C. and Duncan, B. (2001) 'Re-appraising HIV testing among Scottish gay men: the impact of new HIV treatments', *Journal of Health Psychology*, 6, 6, 665–78.

Foucault, M. (1982) *Discipline and punish: the birth of the prison* (Harmondsworth: Penguin).

—— (1988) 'Technologies of the self', in L. Martin, H. Gutman and P. Hutton (eds), *Technologies of the self: a seminar with Michel Foucault* (Amherst: University of Massachusetts Press).

Global HIV Prevention Working Group (2007) *Bringing HIV prevention to scale: an urgent global priority*.www.globalhivprevention.org/pdfs/PWG-HIV_prevention_report_FINAL.pdf (Seattle, WA: Bill and Melinda Gates Foundation and Kaiser Family Foundation), 19 November 2008.

Green, G. and Smith, R. (2004) 'The psychosocial and health care needs of HIV-positive people in the United Kingdom following HAART: a review', *HIV Medicine*, 5, Supplement 1, 1–46.

Health Protection Agency (2008) *HIV in the United Kingdom: 2008 Report* (London: Health Protection Agency).

Herdt, G. (2001) 'Stigma and the ethnographic study of HIV: problems and prospects', *AIDS and Behaviour*, 5, 2, 141–9.

Hyden, L. (1997) 'Illness and narrative', *Sociology of Health and Illness*, 19, 1, 48–69.

Kennedy, C., O'Reilly, K., Medley, A. and Sweat, M. (2007) 'The impact of HIV treatment on risk behaviour in developing countries: a systematic review', *AIDS Care*, 19, 6, 707–20.

Persson, A., Race, K. and Wakeford, E. (2003) 'HIV health in context: negotiating medical technology and lived experience', *Health: An Interdisciplinary Journal for the Social Study of Health, Illness and Medicine*, 7, 4, 397–415.

Porco, T., Martin, J., Page-Shafer, K., Cheng, A., Charlebois, E., Grant, R. and Osmond, D. (2004) 'Decline in HIV infectivity following the introduction of highly active antiretroviral therapy', *AIDS*, 18, 81–8.

Race, K. (2001) 'The undetectable crisis: changing technologies of risk', *Sexualities*, 4, 2, 167–89.

Rofes, E. (1998) *Dry bones breathe: gay men creating post-AIDS identities and cultures* (New York: Harrington Park Press).

Rose, N. (2007) *The politics of life itself: Biomedicine, power, and subjectivity in the twenty-first century* (Princeton: Princeton University Press).

Rosenbrock, R., Dubois-Arber, F., Moers, M., Pinell, P., Schaeffer, D. and Setbon, M. (2000) 'The normalisation of AIDS in Western European countries', *Social Science and Medicine*, 50, 1607–29.

Rosengarten, M., Imrie, J., Flowers, P., Davis, M. and Hart, G. (2004) 'After the euphoria: HIV medical technologies from the perspective of their prescribers', *Sociology of Health and Illness*, 26, 5, 575–96.

Rosengarten, M., Race, K. and Kippax, S. (2001) *'Touch wood, everything will be OK': gay men's understandings of clinical markers in sexual practice* (Sydney: National Centre in HIV Social Research).

Rosenstock, I. (1974) 'Historical origins of the Health Belief Model', *Health Education Monographs*, 2, 4, 328–35.

Sheon, N. and Crosby, M. (2004) 'Ambivalent tales of HIV disclosure in San Francisco', *Social Science and Medicine*, 58, 2105–18.

Squire, C. (2007) *HIV in South Africa: Talking about the big thing* (London: Routledge).

Stephenson, J., Imrie, J., Davis, M., Mercer, C., Copas, A., Black, S., Hart, G., Davidson, O. and Williams, I. (2003) 'Is use of anti-HIV therapy among gay men associated with increased risk of transmission of HIV infection?' *Sexually Transmitted Infections*, 79, 1, 7–10.

Watney, S. (2000) *Imagine hope: AIDS and gay identity* (London: Routledge).

Notes

1. Interviews from Sex, Health and Anti-Retroviral Project (SHARP) are identified by '1'. Interviews conducted as part of my doctoral research are signified '2'. All names used are pseudonyms.

8
Engaging in a Culture of Barebacking: Gay Men and the Risk of HIV Prevention

Kane Race

Introduction

In his book *Autopornography*, the HIV-positive gay pornstar, writer and sex advocate Scott O'Hara gives a frank and amiable account of his sexual experience during the first phase of the AIDS epidemic in North America (O'Hara, 1997a). He describes periods of abstinence, of limiting his sexual practice to certain acts (both alone and with particular partners), of using condoms for anal sex (on one occasion he describes this as 'kinky' and 'hot') and also of unprotected sex. He describes times when he had no libido at all, some of which coincide with periods of illness, and he describes a time after 1994 when his libido returns, when he realises 'there were other HIVers out there with whom I didn't need to worry about transmission; men who didn't worry about isolating bodily fluids' (1997a: 129). Despite his upfront sexual manner and sexual articulacy, O'Hara relates how he found it difficult to raise the subject of AIDS with potential sex partners, such that he'd 'essentially given up sex rather than learn[ed] to discuss it' (1997a: 127). In 1994, he gets an 'HIV+' tattoo on his left bicep (which he refers to as the most visible spot on his body save his forehead) and surrounds it with a 'tasteful little circlet of swimming spermatozoa'. These steps are taken in an attempt to ensure that the sex he has is safe or at least better informed with respect to HIV transmission. For example, on one occasion he describes a sexual encounter with a 'redneck' where he avoids doing anything risky (even oral sex) because it is too dark to see his tattoo. He suggests they jerk each other off in a scene he describes as 'really exciting' (1997a: 200).

Although not all gay men are pornstars or poets, O'Hara's thinking here is typical of the concerns and innovations expressed by many HIV positive gay men.[1] He takes care not to put HIV negative men at risk, and because of his preference for sex without condoms he tries to ensure his sexual partners are other HIV positive men. He describes the risk of sexually transmitted infections and 'possibly other things that are transmissible among HIVers too', but he places little emphasis on these possibilities. 'I assume my partner has the same deductive facilities that I have so I grant him the right to make his own decisions about what precautions he thinks are appropriate' (1997a: 201). O'Hara is alert to the way in which risk and health discourses can be used to naturalise and promote certain moral regimes. At one point, he voices his suspicion that the medical profession's fixation on these dangers 'has more to do with its longstanding distaste for gay sex than on scientific research. You know: Anal Sex – Icky! Dirty!'. Believing some doctors to be 'only too happy to make whatever judgments they can to stop people from having dirty, messy sex', he suggests 'people just need to learn what their own personal safety guidelines are. I doubt the medical profession will offer much realistic help along those lines, so it's up to us to use our noggins' (1997a: 202).

Elsewhere however these risks play a more constitutive role in O'Hara's erotic negotiations with other HIV positive men: 'Nowadays when I make an agreement with a man that we'll fuck uncovered, it's an extreme declaration of trust, knowing that there are potentially lethal diseases that we could be passing back and forth – crypto, meningitis, hepatitis – and we think it's worth the risk.' Though he reports only four instances of this sort of occasion, 'each time stands out, diamond sharp, in my memory, more because of the trust shared than because the sex was extra special' (1997a: 202).[2] Without particularly wishing to object to these instances, it is worth observing that if the stakes of intimacy can be raised in this way it would seem the risks have made some impression.

O'Hara's account is a valuable record of some of the ways gay men have negotiated different and sometimes contradictory formations of sex, infection, risk, responsibility and intimacy. He provides a candid and unapologetic account of the variable positions in which he finds himself as a gendered subject of medical, sexual and romantic discourses. Perhaps what is most confronting in O'Hara's writings for those concerned with HIV prevention is his refusal to subordinate his self-esteem to the prerogatives of HIV prevention. While he never endorses recklessness on the part of HIV positive individuals, he is not prepared to let public health imperatives determine his self-conception as a gay man with a particular relation to HIV.

> I've become somewhat notorious, over the past year, for my positions on HIV. To put it briefly as possible: I can't quite believe it's a curse.

> I'm not trying to out-Louise Ms. Hay, but in my life, AIDS has been an undeniable blessing. It woke me up to what was important; it let me know that NOW was the time to do it. And – this is the part that upsets people – it also gives me the freedom to behave 'irresponsibly'. I look at the HIV negative people around me, and I pity them. They live their lives in constant fear of infection: mustn't do this, mustn't do that, mustn't take risks. They can't see past that simple 'avoidance of infection', which has come to be their ultimate goal. They believe that AIDS = death sentence. Well, I'm sorry, but I was quite possibly infected in 1981, and I'm in pretty good health 15 years later. If that's a death sentence, I guess life in a prison of negativity sounds a lot worse. My life is so much more carefree than theirs, so much more 'considered', that I shake my head and count myself lucky to have been infected. Risk taking is the essence of life, and people who spend their entire lives trying to eliminate risk from their lives are ... well, they're not my kind of people. I know a couple of people who have self-consciously made the decision to seroconvert; I admire them tremendously, because it takes a considerable amount of self-confidence and self-knowledge to make a decision that flies in the face of every medical and journalistic opinion in the world. I applaud this sort of independence. These men are, I might add, some of the most inventive sex partners I've been with. No surprise.
>
> (1997a: 129)

It is illustrative of O'Hara's position as a minoritised sexual and medical subject that his sexual practice entails practices of cultural production. In order to create a viable context for his life he found himself contending forces that would keep both homosexuality and the realities of HIV isolated and private. Though he spent most of his career writing, discussing and practicing sex, at the heart of O'Hara's work as a cultural producer is a conviction that there is nothing very special about it. In the preface to *Autopornography* he writes 'sex is really not the all important subject that my writing would seem to imply' though he admits to having had a 'one-string harp for the past decade'.

> All I want is for sex and porn to take their proper places in life, alongside eating and writing letters – enjoyable activities, not for everyone perhaps, but normal, beneficial, and quite, quite harmless to children. Nothing to get excited about.
>
> (1997a: ix)

For O'Hara, sex is a field of friendly sociability and ordinary belonging. Indeed, when he wants to convey his attitude to sex in his later videos, he does something very unusual in gay porn: he smiles.

In 1993, O'Hara established *Steam* magazine, a publication he edited and billed as a 'Quarterly Journal for Men'. He distributed the first issue free at the March on Washington though later editions came in at a heftier $5.95. The magazine featured accounts of his and other writers' sexual experiences, as well as reports on bathhouses and other areas where gay men meet for sex, and various commentary and writings on sexual matters. Among the contents were regular discussions of HIV issues, though these were not restricted to unexamined rehearsals of public health mantra. The magazine grew to include a literary element, with excerpts of work from writers, scholars and activists such as Samuel R. Delany, Eric Rofes and Pat Califia. *Steam* contributed to what had become a flourishing public culture around sexuality in the US and elsewhere, only one of a multitude of circulars, events, meeting places, conferences, performances, parties and collections that offered alternatives to the authorised construction of sex as rightfully situated in the home, between man and wife, in the context of conjugal intimacy. The magazine was explicit about how it wanted to link sex and public culture.

> We encourage writers, photographers, film-makers, artists, and everyone else to work in the field of sexual expression – not because it's necessarily about Public Sex, but because the more public our sexuality becomes – via, for instance, artwork that deals with it – the less upset society will be with our 'flaunting' our sex in public.
>
> (O'Hara, 1993)

Like other projects of this sort, the magazine hoped to reverse the damaging disinformation of privacy and shame that produces and suffocates subordinate sexualities. Thus whatever problems one might have with the way O'Hara positions HIV seroconversion in the passage cited at length above (where it appears almost as a rite of passage naturalised by gendered constructions of risk, bravado and independence) one can also appreciate the way he helped activate a public setting in which such issues could be debated and collectively and actively negotiated.

I have opened this chapter with a discussion of Scott O'Hara's work as a way into some of the contemporary dimensions of sex and HIV prevention among gay men. O'Hara's discourse is familiar in terms of a certain approach to sex that one encounters in some urban and non-urban gay cultures in various parts of the world – one that I believe to be of some value. In beginning this essay with O'Hara's work I do not wish to overstate or lionise his celebrity or cast him as exemplary, since to do so would be to frame him in terms of some norm or ideality when what I seek is a more ethical engagement with the corpus of material from which his work is drawn. Indeed I find myself in the curious position of wanting at once to affirm and resist O'Hara's authority. O'Hara was only one of the voices that began to speak and write of the pleasures of unprotected sex at about the time that ART was made available in the West (in 1996).[3] These accounts typically referred to unprotected penetrative sex between HIV positive men, something that is safe with respect to HIV transmission. But because they breached established norms around safe sex and the use of condoms, these declarations were the subject of considerable alarm and were attacked as irresponsible by many critics.

I want to affirm such accounts in the sense that they represent creative and situated negotiations of the relations between sex, HIV risk, experimentation and care. They contribute to a larger project of collective self-improvisation and engagement that has been crucial to the success of HIV prevention, and from which the original invention of 'safe sex' sprang.[4] In attending to the situated experience of sex and risk, accounts such as O'Hara's mobilise lay knowledge in the construction of viable intimate practices that avoid HIV transmission. Rather than positioning 'risk' and 'safety' as practices that are set once and for all, they tackle the more difficult and intensive work of conceiving HIV risk as subject to a relational dynamic that involves intimate negotiation between two or more persons as well as changing technologies and conditions.[5] They approach risk as a matter of subjective responsiveness and interpersonal sense-making rather than regulatory prescription by technocrats. The authority to define risk and safety is wrestled away from medical monopoly and opened up onto a public and popularly accessible sphere. This approach has great value for those who wish to promote some movement around HIV prevention.

But O'Hara's account also illustrates some of the risks of liberal, or neoliberal, modes of self-accounting when it comes to the collective responsibility for HIV prevention. His attempt to make sense of his AIDS diagnosis and reject a patient or victim identity sets off alarm bells for the example it might set to both HIV positive and HIV negative men with respect to HIV prevention. Such alarm has grown to define whole agendas of HIV education in the era of ART, particularly in the US, with materials now routinely depicting the more gruesome aspects of treatment side effects in campaigns that explicitly aim to devalue HIV positive experience in the eyes of the gay public and which sometimes seem to be nothing more than a concerted attempt at re-victimisation. One of the values of O'Hara's account is the way it illustrates how this discourse (of positive self-affirmation) preceded the introduction of ART and drew elements from prior discourses of positive self-empowerment and long-term survivorship. His perspective on risk is embedded within a shared experience of long-term survival that preceded ART but was of course unknown at the beginning of the AIDS crisis. Today, the conflict between discourses of positive self-empowerment and discourses of HIV prevention is aggravated by the improved prospects of living with HIV in the context of ART availability and represents a significant impasse in contemporary gay responses to the epidemic.

Thus apart from the sociological insight and ethical complexity that a consideration of O'Hara's work offers in respect of HIV positive sexual practice, another reason for citing him here is that O'Hara is often associated and sometimes even attributed authorship of a specific valuation of unprotected anal sex known as 'barebacking'. Indeed he comes close to claiming this authority for himself when he says in a 1997 opinion piece that he was 'probably the first person to make a public Declaration of Intent to Engage in Unsafe Sex in a national publication' (O'Hara, 1997b).[6] Barebacking emerged in the context of a series of accounts of this sort that provoked outrage both within and outside the gay press, such that it soon took on the sense of an 'erotically charged, premeditated act' with little reference to the question of serostatus (and in some instances at least a highly sensationalised investment in risk on the part of HIV negative men) (Rofes, 1998).[7] I am interested in the conditions in which self-accounts such as O'Hara's can be taken to amount to a defiant and indiscriminate intentionality with respect to HIV transmission, as well as the sense in which those conditions can be understood as disciplinary.[8] I want to suggest that barebacking can be approached as the outcome of a fractious encounter between public morality and embodied ethics in which the latter were basically misrecognised by the former.[9] O'Hara's is a fortuitous instance because of the ethical care (and also self-regard) that can be found in his sexual practice. By tracking the different forms his discourse takes as it moves from one scene of publicity to another we can see how barebacking takes on a life of its own and how this investment in unprotected anal intercourse depends on an encounter between normative apprehension and a defensive response to this apprehension, such that the desire for condomless sex materialises, if only occasionally, as a defiant intent to have *unsafe* sex. In making what could be regarded as a perfectly viable claim around HIV positive sexual practice, barebacking reached for what is perhaps the most available language to defend a practice under attack: the language of individual rights and entitlements. This had the effect of framing sex as a property or entitlement rather than a relation between people, promoting what some have analysed as a presumptive disregard of the other within barebacking discourse (Adam, 2005). It is O'Hara's defensive, individualised citation of the norm and the way it encourages us to relate to sex as an abstract property or entitlement rather than a relational field that I wish to resist. Thus I propose to use O'Hara's writings and their circulation as an entry point into a broader analysis of the normative conditions in which gay sex involving HIV positive subjects becomes uncovered.

'An Intimacy Previously Missing'

Some insight into these conditions can be gleaned from an article that appeared in the *San Francisco Chronicle* in February 2006, entitled 'The Same Sex Scene: A Serosorting Story' (Heredia, 2006). Despite the inflammatory reaction to barebacking in 1997, an apparent decline in the rate of new infections in San Francisco by 2006 despite increases in so-called 'risk practice'[10] led some authorities to embrace what they call 'serosorting' – the practice of selecting sexual partners on the basis of sharing the same HIV status. This is of course the same practice that people like O'Hara were promoting in the furore over barebacking, though now respectabilised some ten years later with a scientific designation (the bitter irony of which is certainly understated by one man interviewed for this article who says, 'I was doing serosorting before they had a word for it. Now, they're saying it is an effective prevention strategy, which is great.') But where barebacking scandalised by virtue of its apparent association with promiscuity and casual sex, serosorting is normalised by means of a conjugal frame that promises 'an intimacy previously missing'.[11] By paying attention to the terms in which serosorting is endorsed for a mainstream audience we can gain insight into some of the forces that mediate the intelligibility of gay sex as it bears on HIV prevention. What is interesting is that while barebacking and serosorting clearly overlap, and may actually refer to the same practice, they proclaim quite different positions in the field of sexual morality, revealing how risk discourse is filtered through more traditional moral categories. Where barebacking foregrounds desire and sensation, and is not always explicit about the concern for HIV prevention that also informs the practice, serosorting foregrounds prevention and risk avoidance, but promotes an oddly desexualised image.

Serosorting is constructed in the article as a form of mutual support ('leaning on each other') in the context of chronic illness, with the added spin-off of HIV containment. The story opens with a 'waiting room romance', at the clinic where two long-term HIV survivors meet and fall in love. The article usefully frames serosorting in terms of the contemporary pressures that bear on HIV positive subjectivity, with the HIV positive individuals interviewed speaking of the stresses associated with the fear of infecting others, the challenges of disclosing HIV status to new partners, and the advantages of negotiating elements of long-term chronic illness in relation with someone who knows what to expect and who is going through something similar. For these individuals, seroconcordant relations are one way of resolving such concerns. A San Francisco couples therapist is quoted:

> I don't think HIV positive men are hooking up to help the community [...] I think they are doing it so they don't have to use condoms and so they can circumvent that HIV coming-out process. They don't want to have to hide their meds [medications]. Physiologically there are changes in their bodies they can't hide. In serosorting they're looking for somebody who doesn't have issues with these things.

These comments anchor serosorting within contemporary practices of HIV positive subjectification, casting it as a reasonable response to current configurations of risk, responsibility, pleasure, health and new technology. But when serosorting is seized upon as a public HIV prevention strategy, something funny happens. The story quotes interview material from Lee, a 44-year-old part-time usher who 'prefers to only date HIV-positive men because he would rather have sex without condoms'. The emergence of HIV dating sites on the Internet and the high proportion of HIV positive gay men in San Francisco are cited as conditions that enable him to disclose his HIV status easily. The inclusion of Lee is noteworthy because his sex life does not adhere strictly to an ideal of long-term conjugal commitment. But Lee is drawn in the heterosexual imagery of 'dating' ('I exclusively date HIV-positive guys'), and is pictured spending time with his partners engaging in couple-like activities such as 'finding entertainment in the community that is low-cost or free'. Meanwhile, James and Brian, the feature couple of the article, are monogamous. The article probes their intimate life.

> The couple's sex life has evolved. At first they had sex without condoms. But after a couple of years together, [Brian] decided he didn't want to risk giving [James] his strain of the HIV virus, a particularly nasty type that is hard to treat. Instead they enjoy kissing, petting, preening and massaging each other [...] 'To be in love with somebody and having a fulfilling life you're not missing out on anything not having penetrative sex', James said.

The article closes with the couple gently caressing and snuggling on the couch, highlighting their 'matching titanium rings'. 'The only time we're apart is when we're on our way to getting together,' says Brian.

The construction of serosorting in this article brings home the importance of attending to the ways in which practices involving minoritised sex and HIV are normatively grasped. Where barebacking was misrecognised as intentional recklessness such that the practical ethics informing the practice were lost, serosorting is celebrated in conventional terms that invisibilise gay practices and cultures of casual sex. It is telling that the valorisation of serosorting in this piece rests on the ultimate erasure of gay anal sex as well as an invocation of matrimonial norms. A normative investment in segregation also becomes apparent with one interview cited, 'Seroselecting is like choosing somebody who is in the same church, like being Episcopalian or Methodist and wanting to marry an Episcopalian or Methodist .... They just get it, you don't have to explain.' There are times in this discourse when serosorting appears to be nothing more than an intricate device through which gay men might be shepherded into normative modes of relationship, sorted by HIV status. The narrative betrays a certain phobia around the very idea of HIV positive people as actively sexual (see Crimp, 1992). But this characteristic only indicates a more immediate problem for HIV prevention workers who must come up with realistic strategies adapted to the practical contexts in which gay sex occurs. While the discourse of serosorting references a widely accessible (and widely accessed) culture of casual sex, it offers a somewhat sanitised version that does not exactly correspond with the sexual culture in which most 'serosorting' takes place. In all the talk around serosorting there is little attention to the relational or situational contexts of gay sex or their practical contingencies. While it is possible that the apparent anonymity of the Internet may make it easier for some HIV positive men to disclose their status when seeking sex online, it remains the case that disclosure is rare in most of the contexts in which gay casual sex occurs, and there are considerable obstacles and practical difficulties around disclosure for HIV positive gay men.[12] Meanwhile in social research a surprising number of HIV negative men indicate rarely knowingly having sex with an HIV positive partner, an expectation that does not reflect reality, and it seems that few HIV negative men are clued into the sometimes very subtle attempts of HIV positive men to negotiate seroconcordant unprotected sex (many of which do not involve spoken disclosure of HIV status).[13] In this sense, the discourse of serosorting may promote a certain brand of wishful thinking that is much more difficult to effect in practice. While after two decades of AIDS it seems important to find ways in which gay men can safely enjoy unprotected anal sex (including in casual contexts), the uncovering of gay sex within serosorting discourse is premised upon a normative misrecognition of much gay sexual practice and promotes this same misrecognition *within* it, raising its own set of challenges and risks.

The appearance of the Internet in this narrative dramatises some of the paradoxes of normative exposure for HIV positive subjects and brings us back to the discussion of O'Hara. For, while norms of individual responsibility would seem to require that HIV positive subjects advertise their status when seeking sex online, it is just such an advertisement that HIV prevention advocates fret over when they suggest that the Internet 'causes' unsafe sex. In the context of barebacking, the Internet was often said to cause risk by virtue of the visibility it gave to HIV positive sex but in the context of serosorting it has become an icon of responsibility. The terms of risk become identifiable with the terms of responsibility here, insofar as both anticipate some level of abstract self-publicity around HIV. It is noteworthy for example that O'Hara cites national publicity as the context for his 'Declaration of Intent'. The norms of abstract personhood that inhere in the national public sphere lead him to discount the relational or embodied contexts of his practice in favour of an assertion of his individual entitlement.[14] O'Hara's self-disclosure can similarly be understood to involve a certain 'taking' of responsibility. His sexual practice is taken in normative terms to be 'irresponsible' though a more detailed account shows that it is carefully considered. Normative constructions of responsibility work here to undercut ethical relations to the self and others and spectacularise them as risk. At this moment, we can see how risk and responsibility enter into a zone of indistinction for HIV subjects and it becomes apparent that barebacking and serosorting run the same range of risks, alternatively grasped – a major misrecognition of minor practices of corporeal responsibility.[15] Perhaps what needs to be contended with here is the normative infrastructure that turns minor instances of self-disclosure into advertisements.

By considering these media in terms of how they work to construct various public and counterpublic identities and subjectivities, we gain insight into how different risks materialise around HIV and what this has to do with normative publicity. If we consider that bodies only make sense within a disciplinary frame shot through with sex and gender norms, we can ask how a sexed and gendered 'grid of intelligibility' mediates the ways in which various responses to HIV become available,[16] and the difference that different scenes of publicity make to the materialisation of these norms. What happens as various parties strive to make minority practices (of HIV risk but also HIV prevention) normatively intelligible? What distortions, identities, impasses, advantages and compromises ensue and how are they negotiated? The combination of minoritised sexuality, mass abstraction and discipline at play here suggests the need to theorise ways in which experience can be grasped as particular, and particularly shared.[17] I am interested therefore in the question of how to engage with barebacking: how one might engage critically with this body of material without inciting the same defiant charge. I want to perform a different relation to the body of material from which O'Hara's voices are drawn – one that is not confined to the dangerous terms of moral denunciation and liberal celebration. This is essentially a methodological question, and in the next section I consider different ways of knowing HIV risk and the different versions of 'responsibility' they produce.

The disciplinary production of intent to engage in unsafe sex

I stated above that this analysis concerns the normative conditions in which gay sex involving HIV positive subjects becomes uncovered. I meant to suggest the ways in which normative constraints on the representation of gay sex and HIV might be considered to be implicated in the proliferation of barebacking. It bears emphasising at this point however that barebacking is only one of the descriptions that gay men give for unprotected sex and individual 'intention' only one of the explanations. In Australia, for example, education has been conducted on how to ensure safe unprotected sex between HIV negative gay men in regular relationships since 1994 (dubbed 'negotiated safety') in a move that many credit to have undermined much of the appeal of so-called 'barebacking'.[18] Apart from this and similar risk reduction practices, gay men account for unsafe sex in a number of ways: erectile difficulty or frustration with condoms, getting carried away with the moment, slipping up, mistaken assumptions about one's partner's HIV status, desiring greater intimacy or intensity, particular relational dynamics (such as not wanting to compromise the encounter because of the partner's presumed superiority and/or desire for unprotected sex), not knowing how to introduce a condom, being drunk or out of it on drugs, forgetting, an accident, personal turmoil – and this is only the beginning of an interminable list, none of which are necessarily best understood as either 'barebacking' or 'intentional'.

Wanting greater precision in their documentation of the offending practice, social scientists have come to define barebacking more strictly as 'intentional unsafe sex'. But as Gregory Tomso has observed, the move to define barebacking strictly as 'intentional unsafe sex' has had the effect of producing barebacking as a problem of volition and desire and generates an even greater scrutiny and policing of gay men's moral intentions (Tomso, 2004). As it stands, even among self-identified barebackers the most common explanations given for their 'intentions' are wanting to experience greater physical stimulation and wanting to feel emotionally connected to their partner. Only 17% of a sample of HIV negative barebackers from San Francisco gave as their reasons wanting to 'do something taboo or racy' while 22% cited as their motivation 'to take a major risk' (these items were not mutually exclusive) (Mansergh et al., 2002).[19] Admittedly surveys are a blunt instrument when it comes to investigating the complexity of subjective meanings, but it would seem that on this definition the eroticisation of risk counts for only a small portion of self-reported barebacking. The subject of my analysis though is not the actual incidence of eroticised risk in the gay population, which would seem to be limited, but *the processes through which unsafe sex materializes as a matter of defiant intention.* I want to approach eroticized risk as the mainly unrealized potential of normal processes of subjectivation and reification occurring at the intersection of familiar discourses of intimacy and risk.[20] These processes could be understood as disciplinary: they involve the recognition of some level of agency and desire among gay men in the vicinity of risk (e.g. the desire for sex without condoms), a normative confrontation or condemnation of that agency and an individualized or aggravated response to that confrontation. Critically, then, my focus is on the refraction of individual desire through official discourse: the contrary effects of the mechanisms through which gay men are responsibilised.[21] I query the system that would erotically construct gay men as intentional deviates when it comes to HIV transmission.[22] As Tomso observes, one cannot separate out 'media representations' and 'scientific facts' here; the conflation of barebacking with other instances of unprotected sex takes place in both the media and the science (Tomso, 2004). And since HIV is such a dense site of positivist social science, I want to turn now to a consideration of how social science participates in this process of risky responsibilisation.

The study 'Barebacking Among Gay and Bisexual Men in New York City: Explanations for the Emergence of Intentional Unsafe Behaviour' sets out to assess 'the frequency with which gay and bisexual men in New York City engage in intentional unprotected sex, or "barebacking"' (Halkitis, Parsons, and Wilton, 2003). The authors set up their report with exemplary precision. They begin by noting that unprotected anal sex has 'gained momentum' in the last several years 'in part because of relapse from safer sex on the part of gay and bisexual men, but also to [sic.] the increasingly popular behavioural phenomenon of intentional unsafe sex, referred to as "barebacking"' (2003: 351). They acknowledge that 'intentional unsafe anal acts may yield minimal or no risk' of HIV transmission in the context of seroconcordant partnerships: unprotected sex between two people known to be of the same HIV status poses no risk of HIV infection. And they discuss the need, by now registered in the science, to differentiate between 'unintentional' unsafe behaviour and 'the increasingly popular unsafe anal practices, which are "intentional" and/or premeditated', and have become 'colloquially known in the mainstream and academic press as "barebacking"'.

This initial meticulousness bears an ambiguous relation to the study's method, however, which the authors outline as follows:

> Participants were asked to respond to the following questions: I am familiar with the term 'barebacking' as it is used by gay men to describe their sexual behavior. No further definition of the 'barebacking' was provided to participants by the research team as we were interested in individual perceptions of the phenomenon; however, 'barebacking' was clearly identified by the survey as a term related to the sexual practices of gay men. Our previous work has shown that barebacking is typically understood by gay men in NYC to refer to intentional unprotected anal intercourse. If they reported familiarity with the term, participants were then asked to report the number of men with whom they had engaged in bareback sex in the 3 months prior to assessment.
>
> (2003: 353)

This method yields the result that 45.5% of the 448 men familiar with the term barebacking reported engaging in bareback sex with at least one sexual partner in the previous three months[23] – a figure that is considerably higher than the 14% reported in a 2002 San Francisco study that explicitly defined barebacking as 'intentional unprotected anal intercourse with a non-primary partner' (Mansergh et al., 2002).[24] On the basis of these findings and documented increases in HIV sero-conversion, the authors propose that 'intentional unprotected sex is increasing among gay and bisexual men' (Halkitis, Parsons, and Wilton, 2003).

To be fair, the meaning of the term 'barebacking' depends on its usage and circulation. It is not set in time, fixed once and for all. Indeed, the method of this study could be considered to be well attuned to the dynamics of the floating signifier: it is necessary and perhaps important for researchers to investigate everyday perceptions and usages of cultural terms, which, after all, may be much wider and more various than any 'original' definition. It's quite probable, in other words, that the term 'barebacking' has travelled well beyond any initial specification and that it is used loosely by many men by this time to refer to unprotected sex in general. (This might explain the fact that half the sample reported engaging in barebacking – a figure that is closer to rates of unprotected sex in this location). That said, there is a tension here between what the study claims to be doing and what it actually does. In particular, it secretly narrows the definition of the term 'barebacking' even as it casts a wide net around the usage of the term among study participants. Through its prefatory definitional work, the study captures as 'intentional unprotected sex' what may in fact be a considerably more diverse range of practices and occasions. It misrecognises the vernacular of participants as completely identifiable with the scientifically defined terms, and thus encourages the subject of its discourse to misrecognise them too. In this sense, the study does indeed offer a convincing 'Explanation for the Emergence of Intentional Unsafe Behavior', as it claims to in the title: the constitutive and normalising work of HIV social science itself! The research is intimately involved in the misrecognition and materialisation of unprotected gay sex as a matter of intention.

In making this claim my aim is not to write off HIV social research in general, nor these researchers in particular, who certainly make a productive contribution to understandings of HIV risk. Rather, the concern is that this mode of enquiry actually promotes a subtle misrecognition of the contingencies of practice, such that gay men are encouraged to recognise, as a matter of 'intention', something that may in fact be much more variable. This is not to argue that gay men are not accountable for what happens in the various sexual contexts in which they find themselves; rather the point is that this mode of identification encourages a turning away from the material and contingent relations of risk, when what could otherwise be promoted is more careful consideration of them. What is being claimed, then, is that this mode of accountability, the crafting of an intentional individual subject of risk – which is as much a corollary of social scientific practice as it is of wider discourse – does not adequately address the circumstances, the matter at hand.

To explore this point further, let us turn to a valuable discussion of the talk of recently diagnosed HIV positive gay men in Sydney. In a perceptive analysis, Sean Slavin and colleagues discuss the range of accounts of unprotected sex that the participants believe to put them at risk, including an account involving considered practices of risk reduction among serodiscordant partners; an account involving sex with an attractive partner while on the recreational drug ecstasy; an account involving 'not caring what happened' and intense feelings of passion and intimacy; and an account involving wanting to 'make things easy' in the context of a relationship with a positive partner (Slavin, Richters, and Kippax, 2004). As the authors discuss, 'These four men narrate their experience of risk not as a result of an accident or misinformation, but as individual choices, informed about risk. Informed, that is, about the technical principles and "objective" facts of viral transmission.'

> They all claim to have known what they were doing at the time of infection and had made a choice, freely and rationally. They all attempt to distinguish between these principles of choice and any emotional, social and cultural context in which they are situated [...]. There is a sense in all these narratives that participants hold themselves solely responsible for having become infected, that they knew what they were doing. They do not consider that context or other factors beyond their control may have mediated the decisions they were making. Such an acknowledgement would seem to question their belief in themselves as 'in control' – of themselves and their circumstances.
>
> (2004: 45)

The authors treat these characteristics as a feature of the discourse or experience of this 'group' of individuals, but what if we were to approach these features as an effect of the disciplinary grid through which these subjects are encouraged to recognise themselves as subjects?

These accounts are made in the context of open-ended interviews conducted a short time after seroconversion.[25] Participants are referred to the study by their HIV clinician and interviewed by a social researcher, either at home or at a community health centre. It is difficult to say whether the context of a private interview gives the participant more or less opportunity to explore their experience in tentative terms – most likely it differs from time to time. But it is interesting to consider what sort of subject is produced in this specific relational context. It is a subject who is rational and decisional and in control of their circumstances, whose choice with respect to risk exists outside any relational or temporal setting, as the authors discuss (2004: 48). Thus, while participants give fairly fluent accounts of the circumstances that they believe placed them at risk, they also insist, as the authors report, on a rational, choice-making self. In particular, they discount the effects of these circumstances on what they call their 'decisions about risk'.

These accounts can be read as records of a process of subjectivation constrained by certain norms of intelligibility: they give clues to the sort of subject that emerges as a product of authorised discourse. Are these individuals participants in acts of 'intentional unsafe sex'? Only within a disciplinary frame that invites them to recognise themselves as such. While it would be possible to argue for the need for a subject even *more* in control of their circumstances given the event of HIV infection in these instances, it is worth considering that such an approach might actually promote further occlusion of the complex relations that make up sexual lives and sexual practices.

In his study of the discourses of HIV positive men in Toronto who use the language of barebacking to refer to their practice, Barry Adam finds that 'interviews with self-professed barebackers reveal not so much rebellion or transgression as something more prosaic and more consistent with the discourses of government and capital. Not only does the responsibilisation message resonate throughout their own accounts but the larger rhetoric of neoliberalism does as well, of which responsibility talk is a part' (Adam, 2005). Adam's analysis deals only with HIV positive barebackers, who can be expected to bear a mitigated relation to the erotics of risk.[26] He locates barebacking as a personal policy found among some HIV positive men within urban gay community, embedded in a larger context of encountering men who are HIV positive or 'in the know'. As is evident in O'Hara's accounts of his sexual practice, neither the practical morality nor the actual practices of the HIV positive men interviewed 'overtly intend HIV transmission to happen' (2005: 341).[27] But as Adam illustrates, their practice relies on extremely subtle negotiations that HIV negative men are often unaware of and, perhaps more significantly, it does not allow for the complex 'vulnerabilities, emotions and tough dilemmas' that characterise everyday life and sexual interaction (2005: 344).

One of the values of Adam's study is the way it illustrates how the discourse of barebackers is consonant with wider, even dominant, discourses that structure social life and moral reasoning. 'In many ways,' Adam writes, 'these accounts for unsafe sex participate in the moral reasoning widely propagated by government and business today that constructs each as a self-interested individual who must take responsibility for himself in a marketplace of risks. It is perhaps also a particularly masculine discourse in its evocation of norms of competitive individualism' (2005: 340). However, unlike so many accounts of gay life circulating even in 'progressive' circles today, Adam does not hold gay men up as 'exemplars' of neoliberal ideology, but rather remains alive to the virtualities of subject formation. He suggests that 'neoliberal discourse is not totalising nor does it capture the subjectivity of these men in a fundamental way', pointing to competing discourses 'drawn from romance, masculine adventure, gay solidarity, communitarianism, and so on, that can come to the fore, according to circumstance' (2005: 345). By appealing to gay men to take care of other men '(instead of simply defending themselves against other men)', he locates his critique within a tradition of gendered counterpractice. 'It would be an appeal that would run against leading ideologies in circulation in our society today but one that would likely have considerable resonance among men whose sexual pursuits are often linked with the desire to love and be loved by other men' (2005: 345). Especially useful in this regard is the way Adam's methodology undercuts some of the epistemological and technical commitments of neoliberalism. He recognises and documents the moral intentions of his subjects but also finds ways of suggesting that a mere focus on *intentions* is not the end of a practical response. In this sense, his analysis works in precisely the opposite direction to the discourses I have been discussing, which totalise the question of intention while ignoring the circumstances of prevention. Rather than debunking neoliberal ideologies in a familiar critical style, Adam recognises their sedimentation in the embodied experience of those whom he engages and gestures towards other possibilities and tendencies. The ethical sensibilities of participants can thus become involved in a wider querying of normative terms. Insofar as it gestures towards the processual nature of subject formation, and emphasises the constitutive work of broader political technologies in these processes, I believe this mode of enquiry offers a better basis for an ethical engagement with barebacking.

Conclusion

In this essay I have been concerned with the disciplinary technologies through which gay men are made into subjects of HIV prevention. I have argued that in making themselves, and being made, into subjects of HIV prevention, gay men may be led to interpret certain of their sexual activities and desires as intentional deviance with respect to HIV risk, and this leads to a misrecognition of the preventive possibilities of their practice. This process can be understood as an effect, in part, of the disciplinary grid through which HIV subjects are currently produced. If barebacking understands itself as an eroticisation of the transgression of public health and gay community norms, then it is necessary for those who are concerned with HIV prevention to work against the reification of those norms by adopting more flexible mode of attentiveness to the circumstances of sex, pleasure and HIV transmission.

In recent years various attempts have been made to decipher the meanings of barebacking. In turn psychological and anthropological, these efforts purport to approach barebacking as an exotic or foreign subculture with its own set of meanings, presumed unified and coherent. But perhaps the presumption of unity and coherence is a mistake. Even the most brilliant of these readings tend to downplay the importance of certain distinctions that exist: between unprotected sex and HIV transmission, between serodiscordance and seroconcordance, between fantasy and practice. These distinctions are highly material, both for purposes of HIV prevention, and for the participants themselves, for whom HIV prevention is often also a possible source of concern. In contrast to this approach, here I have been concerned to situate barebacking – both the practice and the desire – in terms of the knowledge practices that attend and produce it. From this perspective, sex without condoms is multiple. Sometimes it is produced as barebacking. Sometimes it is produced as serosorting, or 'negotiated safety'. Sometimes it is produced as an erotic transgression of gay community and public health norms. At other times it may be produced as an erotic expression of ingenuity and survival. How it is enacted is a question that is inseparable from the knowledge practices that apprehend and produce it. From this perspective, sex without condoms is a prime example of what Annemarie Mol has called 'ontological politics' – a term that has been coined to describe the active shaping of reality through different knowledge practices (Mol, 2002). It is multiply enacted, and those who are concerned with HIV prevention are charged with the task of creating conditions in which it might be enacted without occasioning HIV transmission. Part of this project involves understanding safe sex as a dynamic practice that takes different forms in different historical and cultural contexts (see Race, 2003; 2009). To this end, I have found an analytic distinction between normative morality and practical ethics a useful way of bringing certain innovations in HIV prevention to wider attention.

References

Adam, Barry D. 2005. 'Constructing the Neoliberal Sexual Actor: Responsibility and Care of the Self in the Discourse of Barebackers'. *Culture, Health & Sexuality*, 7:333–46.

Agamben, Giorgio. 1995. *Homo Sacer: Sovereign Power and Bare Life*. Translated by D. Heller-Roazen. Stanford: Stanford University Press.

Berlant, Lauren. 1997. *The Queen of America Goes to Washington City: Essays on Sex and Citizenship*. Durham/London: Duke University Press.

Berlant, Lauren and Michael Warner. 1998. 'Sex in Public'. *Critical Inquiry*, 24:547–66.

—— 2004. *Undoing Gender*. New York: Routledge.

Crimp, D. 1992. 'Portraits of People with AIDS' in *Cultural Studies* (eds) L. Grossberg, C. Nelson, and P. Triechler. London/New York: Routledge.

Escoffier, Jeffrey. 1999. 'The Invention of Safer Sex: Vernacular Knowledge, Gay Politics and HIV Prevention'. *Berkley Journal of Sociology*, 43:1–30.

Foucault, Michel. 1977. *Discipline and Punish: The Birth of the Prison*. Translated by A. Sheridan. London: Penguin.

—— 1982. 'The Subject and Power'. pp. 208–26 in *Michel Foucault: Beyond Structuralism and Hermeneutics*, (eds) H. Dreyfus and P. Rabinow. New York: Harvester Wheatsheaf.

—— 1984. *The Use of Pleasure: The History of Sexuality 2*, vol. 2. Translated by R. Hurley. London: Penguin.

Halkitis, Perry, J. Parsons, and L. Wilton. 2003. 'Barebacking among Gay and Bisexual Men in New York City: Explanations for the Emergence of Intentional Unsafe Behavior'. *Archives of Sexual Behaviour*, 32:351–7.

Halperin 2007. *What Do Gay Men Want: An Essay on Sex, Risk and Subjectivity*. Ann Arbor: University of Michigan Press.

Heredia, Christopher 2006. 'The Same Sex Scene'. *San Francisco Chronicle*, 12 February.

Kinder, P. 1996. 'A New Prevention Education Strategy for Gay Men: Responding to the Impact of AIDS on Gay Men's Lives' in *XI International AIDS Conference*. Vancouver.

Kippax, S. 2002. 'Negotiated Safety Agreements among Gay Men'. pp. 1–15 in *Beyond Condoms: Alternative Approaches to HIV Prevention* (eds) A. O'Leary. New York: Kluwer/Plenum Press.

Kippax, Susan and Kane Race. 2003. 'Sustaining Safe Practice: Twenty Years On'. *Social Science and Medicine*, 57:1–12.

Mansergh, G., G. Marks, G. Colfax, R. Guzman, M. Rader, and S. Buchbinder. 2002. '"Barebacking" in a Diverse Sample of Men Who Have Sex with Men'. *AIDS*, 16:653–9.

Mol, Annemarie. 2002. *The Body Multiple: Ontology in Medical Practice*. Durham: Duke University Press.

O'Hara, Scott 1993. 'Steam Gets Culture'. *Steam*, Autumn, p. 146.

—— 1997a. *Autopornography: A Memoir of Life in the Lust Lane*. New York: Harrington Park Press.

—— 1997b. 'Safety First? Risks of Sexual Intimacy'. *The Advocate*, 8 July, p. 9.

Patton, Cindy. 1990. *Inventing AIDS*. New York: Routledge.

Race, Kane. 2003. 'Revaluation of Risk among Gay Men'. *AIDS Education and Prevention*, 15:369–81.

—— 2009. *Pleasure Consuming Medicine: The Queer Politics of Drugs*. Durham: Duke University Press.

Rofes, Eric. 1998. *Dry Bones Breathe: Gay Men Creating Post-AIDS Identities and Cultures*. Binghampton: Harrington Park Press.

Rosengarten, Marsha. 2009. *HIV Interventions: Biomedicine and the Traffic between Information and Flesh*. Washington: University of Washington Press.

Rosengarten, Marsha, Kane Race, and Susan Kippax. 2000. 'Touch Wood, Everything Will Be Okay: Gay Men's Understandings of Clinical Markers in Sexual Practice'. National Centre in HIV Social Research, University of New South Wales, Sydney.

Sheon, N and G Crosby. 2004. 'Ambivalent Tales of HIV Disclosure in San Francisco'. *Social Science and Medicine*, 58:2105–18.

Slavin, S., J. Richters, and S. Kippax. 2004. 'Understandings of Risk among HIV Seroconverters in Sydney'. *Health, Risk & Society*, 6:39–52.

Stephenson, Niamh and D. Papdopoulos. 2006. *Analysing Everyday Experience: Social Research and Political Change*. London: Palgrave Macmillan.

Tomso, Gregory. 2004. 'Bug Chasing, Barebacking, and the Risks of Care'. *Literature and Medicine*, 23:88–111.

Van de Ven, Paul, P. Rawstorne, J. Crawford, and S. Kippax. 2001. 'Facts and Figures: 2000 Male out Survey'. National Centre in HIV Social Research.

Warner, Michael. 1999. *The Trouble with Normal: Sex, Politics and the Ethics of Queer Life*. Cambridge, MA: Harvard University Press.

—— 2002. *Publics and Counterpublics*. New York: Zone Books.

Notes

This chapter is a shortened and slightly revised version of "Engaging in a Culture of HIV Prevention: Gay Men and the Risk of HIV Prevention", first published in *Gendered Risks*, edited by Kelly Hannah-Moffat and Pat O'Malley (Oxon: Routledge-Cavendish, 2007) pp. 99–126. I thank Routledge-Cavendish for permission to reprint here. I would also like to thank David Halperin, Susan Kippax, Marsha Rosengarten and Niamh Stephenson for reading and commenting on earlier versions of this article and Adrian Kerr for enduring the writing of it.

1. For qualitative evidence to this effect, see Barry Adam's rigorous analysis in Adam, Barry D. 2005. 'Constructing the Neoliberal Sexual Actor: Responsibility and Care of the Self in the Discourse of Barebackers'. *Culture, Health & Sexuality*, 7:333–46. An early study of practices of safety outside the condom code exists in Rosengarten, Marsha, Kane Race, and Susan Kippax. 2000. 'Touch Wood, Everything Will Be Okay: Gay Men's Understandings of Clinical Markers in Sexual Practice'. National Centre in HIV Social Research, University of New South Wales, Sydney. See also [Race 2003].
2. Elsewhere he writes of his HIV+ partner 'When I tell Chris – lovingly – that I want to feel him shoot inside me, unprotected, it indicates a level of trust, of cohesion, that I don't think is achievable when both partners are primarily concerned with preventing the exchange of bodily fluids'. O'Hara, Scott 1997b. 'Safety First? Risks of Sexual Intimacy'. *The Advocate*, 8 July, p. 9.
3. ART, or HAART (Highly active ART) were terms coined to denote combination therapy involving a new class of drugs, protease inhibitors, publicised at the 1996 International AIDS Conference in Vancouver. Where it is made available (it still reaches only small section of the world's HIV-infected population), ART is celebrated as converting HIV/AIDS from a fatal condition to a chronic manageable illness.
4. Kippax and Race 2003, Halperin 2007 and Race 2009 See Escoffier, J. 1999. 'The Invention of Safer Sex: Vernacular Knowledge, Gay Politics and HIV Prevention'. *Berkley Journal of Sociology*, 43:1–30; Patton, Cindy. 1990. *Inventing AIDS*. New York: Routledge.
5. For a highly innovative conception of the relation between HIV medical technologies and sexual practice see Rosengarten, Marsha (2009). *HIV Interventions Biomedicine and the Traffic between Information and Flesh*. Washington: University of Washington Press.
6. This piece appears in the mainstream gay publication *The Advocate* and refers to a 1995 editorial in *Steam* magazine, 'Exit the Rubberman', which thematically resembles the passage quoted at length above, though it adopts even more strident tones. I am grateful to the late Eric Rofes for finding me a copy of 'Exit the Rubberman'.
7. Rofes provides a vital and engaged account of this moment in the North American context.
8. I use this term in Foucault's sense to refer to the process, peculiar to modern societies, of distributing behaviour around a given norm and producing it in terms of normal or abnormal individuality. I want to emphasise the individualising force of this process of subject formation, whereby subjects are led to assess their individuality against norms of HIV prevention (here, the condom code). See Foucault, Michel. 1977. *Discipline and Punish: The Birth of the Prison*. Translated by A. Sheridan. London: Penguin.
9. On the distinction between ethics and the normative moral code see [Foucault 1984]. For an application of this distinction to gay men's sexual practice in the interests of HIV prevention see [Race 2003]. On publicity and the potential distortion of minority sexualities see [Warner 2002].
10. That is risk, as reified in the practice of unprotected anal intercourse.
11. The byline of the article reads: 'Dating within the HIV positive or negative population has reduced the HIV infection rate in San Francisco. It also allows for an intimacy previously missing.' See [Berlant 1997] and [Berlant and

Warner 1998] on the politics and institutions of intimacy in the neoconservative US.

12. Even in San Francisco. See Sheon, N and G Crosby. 2004. 'Ambivalent Tales of HIV Disclosure in San Francisco'. *Social Science and Medicine*, 58:2105–18.
13. For a lucid illustration of this point, see Adam, Barry D. 2005. 'Constructing the Neoliberal Sexual Actor: Responsibility and Care of the Self in the Discourse of Barebackers'. *Culture, Health & Sexuality*, 7:333–46. His observations are borne out by survey data in Australia. See Van de Ven, Paul, P. Rawstorne, J. Crawford, and S. Kippax. 2001. 'Facts and Figures: 2000 Male out Survey'. National Centre in HIV Social Research. 36–7.
14. For more on the risks and paradoxes of mass abstraction for minority subjects see Warner, Michael. 2002. *Publics and Counterpublics*. New York: Zone Books and Berlant, Lauren. 1997. *The Queen of America Goes to Washington City: Essays on Sex and Citizenship*. Durham/London: Duke University Press.
15. On zones of indistinction and the politics of exposure see Agamben, Giorgio. 1995. *Homo Sacer: Sovereign Power and Bare Life*. Translated by D. Heller-Roazen. Stanford: Stanford University Press.
16. My use of the term 'grid of intelligibility' is informed by the recent work of Judith Butler, who uses it to show how processes of self-reporting and self-understanding are structured by social norms, in particular sex and gender norms. Butler, Judith. 2004. *Undoing Gender*. New York: Routledge. Butler situates the concept in relation to processes of recognition and self-recognition: 'Indeed, if we consider that human bodies are not experienced without recourse to some ideality, some frame for experience itself, and that this is true for the experience of one's own body as it is for experiencing another, and if we accept that that ideality and frame are socially articulated, we can see how it is that embodiment is not thinkable without a relation to a norm, or set of norms' (28). The value of this approach is that it directs attention to the conditions in which subjecthood and identity is produced. It asks that we examine the interplay of practice and recognition, and see how social norms mediate and structure that process.
17. I thank Niamh Stephenson for pressing this point in her many discussions with me on this issue. See Stephenson, Niamh and D. Papdopoulos. 2006. *Analysing Everyday Experience: Social Research and Political Change*. London: Palgrave Macmillan.
18. See Kippax, S. 2002. 'Negotiated Safety Agreements among Gay Men'. pp. 1–15 in *Beyond Condoms: Alternative Approaches to HIV Prevention*, (eds) A. O'Leary. New York: Kluwer/Plenum Press. The phrase 'negotiated safety' was first coined by [Kinder 1996].
19. Interestingly, these explanations were less pertinent for HIV positive barebackers, of whom only 10% and 7% cited them respectively.
20. See the discussion of how risk discourse intensifies intimacy and eroticism in O'Hara's discourse above, cited in the third paragraph of this chapter.
21. This can be theorised in Foucauldian terms as an operation of power that 'applies itself to immediate everyday life which categorises the individual, marks him by his own individuality, attaches him to his own identity, imposes a law of truth on him which he must recognise and which others

have to recognise in him,' whereby barebackers identify the excitement of sex without condoms as the truth of their identity. Foucault, Michel. 1982. 'The Subject and Power'. pp. 208–26 in *Michel Foucault: Beyond Structuralism and Hermeneutics*, (eds) H. Dreyfus and P. Rabinow. New York: Harvester Wheatsheaf.

22. As Tomso has written, 'bug chasing and barebacking exist as phenomena largely because of what Foucault would call the constitutive, disciplinary operation of scientific, activist, and popular discourses about them. That is to say that those who are currently investigating and writing about these phenomena, as much so if not more than the men whose sexual lives are the subjects of these investigations, are epistemologically accountable for the emergence of bug chasing and barebacking as social "problems"(2004: 89). I would add ontologically.
23. This figure represents 60.9% of the HIV positive respondents and 41.8% of the HIV negative respondents, and is inclusive of unprotected sex between men of the same HIV status (which in fact accounts for the majority of instances).
24. It should be noted that the latter study excludes instances of 'intentional unprotected sex' that have taken place within a primary partnership, which the Halkitis study may conceivably include.
25. Between two weeks and several months. Participants are asked to recount the event(s) they believe led to their infection. The accounts mentioned differ from other participants in the study who believed they had followed moral prescriptions regarding sexual morality and are taken by surprise (rather than experiencing themselves as 'in control' subjects).
26. See, for example, the findings from Mansergh et al. discussed above in note 29. In barebacking fantasies on the Internet, the HIV positive role is usually constructed in terms of 'gift-giving' and 'seeding' – metaphors that have less to do with eroticised risk than with community initiation, belonging and some version of a familiar mythology of intimacy, fertility and procreation.
27. Many participants speak of modifying their practice in the direction of safety upon learning of a partner's HIV negative status, and the study includes accounts of the considerable lengths some men go to when they discover a mistake has been made.

9

HIV Pre-exposure Prophylaxis (PrEP) and the Complexities of Biomedical Prevention: Ontological Openness and the Prevention Assemblage

Marsha Rosengarten and Mike Michael

Introduction

In this chapter we examine the challenges identified in the development of a pharmaceutically based oral HIV pre-exposure prophylaxis referred to as PrEP, and how the issues raised in the course of early and current clinical trials enable a rethinking of the possibilities for HIV prevention. Drawing on an ethnographic study of PrEP involving new theoretical developments in the field of Science and Technology Studies (STS) we pose PrEP and HIV prevention, more generally, as an assemblage that is ontologically open rather than, as more usually conceived, made up of stable and distinct objects: drugs, bodies, condoms and virus. Biomedical and non-biomedical forms of prevention lend themselves to the concept of assemblage as the latter conveys a dynamic involving inter-relationships between heterogeneous phenomena. The processual nature of this inter-relationality produces an open system of 'complex becoming and multiple determinations' (Venn, 2006: 107) through which the potential to intercept an unwanted form of inter-relationality – the achievement of viral viability or, put more simply, infection – can take place.

Although we preface this chapter with the caveat that our work is, at this stage, exploratory and for the most part intended to serve as a provocation rather than a complete methodological alternative, our broader aim is to continue to adapt new and novel conceptions in the area of STS to the field of HIV. Our ethnographic study is the first part of this project which, to date, has been focused on the relationship between ethics, science and HIV prevention in response to the worrying phenomenon of increasing HIV infections. During late 2007 and intermittently during 2008, we interviewed 20 scientific stakeholders in PrEP while also examining the role of published literature including the use of internet sites. Our interviews included principal investigators and associate investigators of PrEP trials being conducted in the US, Thailand, Peru, Ecuador, Botswana as well as trials planned for South Africa, Tanzania, Malawi, Kenya, Zimbabwe. They also included some of the investigators involved in the trials halted in Cambodia and Cameroon. Other interviewees were bench scientists, trial advocates and community activists. Each respondent was invited to comment on what they perceived to be the promise and challenges of PrEP. In this text, respondents have been anonymised.

PrEP

PrEP is currently conceived or imagined as similar to the contraceptive pill or to an anti-malaria pill. It consists of 'one pill a day' made up of the HIV antiretroviral drug Tenofovir which, in some instances, is combined with Emtricitabine and called Truvada.[1] Both Tenofovir and Emtricitabine are used as part of HIV antiretroviral combination treatments (ART). The two drugs are manufactured by the pharmaceutical company Gilead Sciences and have been selected as a possible PrEP because of favourable drug resistance profiles and anticipated few side effects when compared to other antiretroviral drugs. For readers unfamiliar with antiretroviral drugs, it will be important to know that the key concerns about these drug types are their potential to engender viral resistance and also the possibility of life threatening or, lesser but still worrying, life disruptive toxic 'side-effects'. In reference to PrEP, the likelihood that it will be only 'partially effective', in turn, raises the issue of viral resistance which could develop with infections occurring under conditions equivalent to sub-optimal therapy. 'Partial effectiveness' is anticipated if coverage is uneven across a population and/or within an individual body, especially but not only because people may forget to take their pills. Different strains of HIV may also affect PrEP's effectiveness. Another possibility is that PrEP could be more effective against one sort of exposure than another, for instance, it might be effective in protecting against vaginal rather than anal exposure (AVAC, 2005). Compounding the medical concerns is a broader concern with sexual 'disinhibition', that is, awareness by HIV affected communities of a possible form of PrEP may reduce concern about HIV risk and result in a decline in condom use, leading to increases in infections. 'Disinhibition' – as declines in condom use have been interpreted (Grant et al., 2005; AVAC, 2008) – is especially worrisome if the level of partial effectiveness warrants continued use of condoms. As a type of worst case scenario, 'partial effectiveness' means that PrEP could produce not just more people who are infected but, also, more drug-resistant virus with the effect of undermining treatment options. The complicated range of potential problems – set out here based on stakeholder accounts – raises questions about whether or how this chemo-prophylaxis is appropriate for prevention purposes in otherwise 'healthy' HIV *negative* bodies.

Despite the potential problems, the rationale for considering PrEP appears strong. Below are key reasons put forward by policy analysts and advocacy groups:

(1) 2.5 million people are becoming infected each year worldwide, despite existing prevention technologies, namely condoms and clean needles (UNAIDS/WHO, 2007).
(2) There is still no significant advance producing an HIV vaccine and topical microbicides (vaginal and anal barrier gels or creams) are still in early stages of development (AVAC, 2008).
(3) There is powerful evidence that ARVs can prevent infection from mother-to-child during pregnancy and labour (MTCP); and also may prevent infection post exposure (PEP) if a course is commenced within 72 hours of needle stick injury or sexual intercourse.[2]
(4) There have been some relatively convincing animal studies of PrEP (AVAC, 2008).
(5) In the absence of a vaccine, it could be beneficial to have another form of biomedical technology that can be taken on a regular basis and not dependent on implementation at the time of sexual intercourse (the case with condoms).
(6) If found efficacious through randomised clinical trials (RCTs), existing licensing for Tenofovir and Emtricitabine mean that PrEP could be made available immediately.

On the basis of the above rationale for PrEP, a series of Phase II/III randomised PrEP clinical trials have been planned and some are underway in sub-Saharan Africa, Asia, South America and the US.[3] Most notable from this spread of continents and regions and, indeed, one of the drivers of this paper is that, with the exception of the US, all trials are in low and middle income countries where the provision of health care and the availability of ART is significantly lacking in contrast to the country location of trial sponsor and principal researchers (mainly

US but also Australia).[4] Important also to point out is that unlike many other pharmaceutical trials, the sponsorship of those for PrEP is through public and/or philanthropic sources and not commercial interests. So far, the trials have been funded through the US Centers for Disease Control and Prevention (CDC), the US Agency for International Development (USAID), the US National Institutes of Health (NIH) and the Bill & Melinda Gates Foundation (AVAC, 2008). The only direct involvement of Gilead Sciences is as a provider of the drugs and the placebo, free of cost for the trials. Further, Gilead has made provision for the drugs to be made available at 'cost' to populations in low and middle income countries, if they are found to be effective as a prophylaxis (Paxton et al, 2007; Singh and Mills 2005).

Our interest in PrEP was initially invoked by a controversy that emerged in response to three of the planned trials. The controversy was first aired internationally at the XV International AIDS Conference, Bangkok, where a protest was staged outside the Gilead stand by members of the Cambodian Women's Network for Unity (Mills et al., 2006). It also took a textual form on websites where media statements were released by activist groups and, later, researchers, advocates and bioethicists responded to these by placing other material on websites and by producing a small number of refereed journal articles (Grant et al., 2005; Jintarkanon et al., 2005; Mills et al., 2005, 2006; Page-Shafer et al., 2005; Singh and Mills, 2005; The Thai AIDS Treatment Action Group, 2004). Although we do not intend to rehearse the controversy, we do want to convey something of its flavour as it has mobilised an ensuing debate which, in itself, provides some of the ground on which we will begin to introduce an alternative methodological approach. That is to say, the material generated in the wake of initial controversy is an important source of the complexity that comprises PrEP and that, we, go on to show, may be usefully conceived as a *dynamic processual* or assemblage involving considerably more actors – human and non-human – than a conventional bioethical account of research and researcher.

Public airings of PrEP trials and the shortcomings of bioethics

In December 2004, a statement was released by six Thai-based activist groups in anticipation of a scheduled PrEP trial seeking to enrol injecting drug users (IDUs) at risk of HIV infection for whom clean needles and syringes would not be provided as part of the trial. The statement made reference to paragraph 29 of the Declaration of Helsinki which declares that a placebo-controlled trial should only be used in the absence of existing prophylactic (in this instance, clean needles and syringes), diagnostic and therapeutic methods. This point was followed by an account of the political situation in Thailand where access to HIV antiretroviral therapies (ART) for HIV positive IDUs may be conditional on quitting injecting drug use. Other concerns expressed in the statement included the lack of guaranteed access to PrEP after one year, post the trial, if the biotechnology is found to be effective and, also, a general lack of consultation with trial-affected community groups (Thai AIDS Treatment Action Group et al., 2004; Jintarkanon et al., 2005). In response, the trial organisers initially defended the trial design saying that it accorded with Thai government prohibition on the free distribution of needles and noted that bleach was provided for sterilising needles for their reuse. They also pointed out that clean needles and syringes can be purchased legally from local pharmacies (Mills et al., 2005: 1404–5). However, by agreeing to Thai government policy and not providing proven prophylaxes for trial participants, the trial organisers were liable to accusations that they were colluding with the Thai government in the making of high risk. Indeed advocates for those involved in the trial and for other IDUs pointed out that the US researchers were consenting to unfair and discriminatory policies that arguably contravene human rights arguments.[5] Results from this trial were expected in 2009, at the time of this article going to press it is still underway without provision of clean needles and syringes.

In January 2005, Irin News, within the UN Office for the Coordination of Humanitarian Affairs, reported that the government of Cameroon had stated that it might stop clinical trials of PrEP planned for testing on 400 female sex workers. This followed allegations that the women were receiving inadequate counselling and that there were no guarantees that medical care would be available to those who became infected during the trial. Soon after, the trial was halted by the government and prolonged negotiations took place. Although the trial was finally agreed to by the government, the sponsor Family Health International made the decision to close it (Mills et al., 2005: 1403).[6] The activities in Cameroon followed the cancellation by the Cambodian government of a PrEP trial planned to take place there with female sex workers. Both Cambodian and Cameroon activists voiced similar objections about counselling and medical care.[7] While lead researchers from the Cambodian trial have since stated that provision was made for counselling and medical care, local activists understood differently. Certainly, it seems, arrangements for the provision of antiretroviral treatment in the long term for trial participants who become HIV infected during the trial, that is, acquired 'intercurrent infection', were unclear (Mills et al., 2006).

The issue of intercurrent infection is recognised as a phenomenon particular to HIV biomedical clinical trials. Although increasingly researchers are committing to ensure the provision of antiretroviral access and this commitment is made more possible as treatment access improves in middle and some low income countries, international agencies such as UNAIDS and WHO see it as outside the researchers' obligations of care to their research subjects. The view of such agencies lags well behind their own recognition that intercurrent infections are necessary to the success of any biomedical prevention trial. The WHO/UNAIDS report '*Treating people with intercurrent infection in HIV prevention trials*', published in 2004 before the advent of PrEP trials, states that the strongest justification for providing antiretroviral drugs for those who do seroconvert during the trial is that 'the occurrence of HIV infection is required in order to demonstrate the efficacy of the prevention intervention' (WHO/UNAIDS, 2004: 4). HIV infections demonstrate the probability that a significant percentage of participants have been exposed to HIV during the period of the trial. Consequently, they form the data against which the candidate or agent can be evaluated for its effectiveness in comparison with the placebo (Bass and Kahn, 2005). However, the same report goes on to complicate the commitment that could follow the recognition by raising a series of questions about, for instance, what level of care should be provided, who is responsible and should a partner receive antiretrovirals at levels comparable with those who were enrolled in the trial (WHO/UNAIDS, 2004: 4). Ultimately, the report leaves the reader with a sense that although the moral commitment is present, the practicalities prevent an internationally standardised ethical commitment. Not surprisingly in the absence of international standardisation, scientific researchers accustomed to the procedures of standardisation find themselves faced with what they understand as an ethical quandary that arises in the asymmetrical relations incurred by what is presumed necessary in scientific research. As MacQueen et al. (2007: 554) put it,

> Epidemiologically, they [people in developing countries] are the people with the greatest need for effective prevention; statistically, they also present the most efficient opportunity to test interventions but the poverty and disempowerment that generate vulnerability to HIV infection also serve as barriers to medical care and services. Thus, the people most appropriate for enrolment [sic] in international HIV

> prevention trials are also the people least likely to have access to HIV treatment and care in their local communities.

In contrast to what is available in the home country of sponsors and lead researchers, a trial participant in a developing country is likely to have significantly less access to health care and medical resources. In turn, their trial-incurred needs may place more pressure on already inadequate familial, local and national resources. Perhaps most indicative of how the vulnerability important to HIV RCTs may be compounded, the presence of a trial bearing the promise of an effective intervention is often debated in terms of whether it will undermine or 'disinhibit' community perceptions of risk. As we mentioned in our introduction, this is a major concern as it is recognised as having the potential to lead to more unsafe practice resulting in increases in infection (AVAC, 2008). As a corollary, the impoverished conditions associated with HIV vulnerability could mean an increase in the number of people with limited or no access to the drugs for treatment.

Given this seeming paradox, public or philanthropically funded HIV researchers consider and enact bioethics through the establishment of Ethical Oversight Committees to monitor the workings of a trial.[8] However, this achieves a general acceptance that the tension in conducting 'offshore' clinical trials is solely about bioethics and these can be addressed through mechanisms additional to the science of the trial. By posing trials as a necessary procedure for the *future* alleviation of the problem of HIV vulnerability, the trial itself is able to be performed at a conceptual distance from the everyday issues of context-affected HIV vulnerability with direct and possibly untapped material consequences. This is not to deny that trials may inform the implementation of a technology such as PrEP.[9] Nor is it to underplay the potential advance in health and medical infrastructure that may follow from the undertaking of a trial. Indeed, the potential available through the import of state-of-the-art-science is, itself, a site of enquiry that may benefit from the argument we make here. Key, though, to any review of the development of HIV prevention – biomedical or otherwise – are the relations that take place through the trial for circumventing the viability of the virus. Although PrEP continues to be enacted by those involved in its development as if distinct from the human and non-human relations that inform it, it is these relations which are the matter of ethics, science and prevention. As we shall show, the activity of these relations can be mapped to evidence prevention as ontologically open and illustrated here through reference to the highly contingent nature of PrEP.

Heterogeneity and multiple functionality

To demonstrate what we mean by suggesting that prevention can be understood as ontologically open and propose this openness as giving rise to multiple functionalities, we now refer to data from our qualitative research to date. Elaborating on PrEP, the following account makes apparent that it is an intensely complex phenomenon comprising relations between numerous heterogeneous entities likely to generate further relations.

> They [trials] use a standard dose but when the dose goes into the person ... there's a couple of different things. There's a variability in drug exposure within each individual. We may see in certain people who have lower exposures to the drugs that perhaps PrEP fails, and then in people who have higher exposures, PrEP is successful. But then there is also the adherence piece. So if people are not as adherent to a regimen – if this is a once a day PrEP regimen – then we may be able to see that with the samples that are being collected over time, and that will change exposure as well. If people aren't being as adherent to their therapy, or to their regimen, then [drug] exposures will be lower in those individuals.
>
> (Respondent 11)

The heterogeneous nature of what determines the efficacy of PrEP against HIV infection gives rise to a dynamic processual. Indeed, in another paper we have proposed that the processual may be understood to produce many PrEPs as 'it' emerges out of and embodies different associations that perform differently (Rosengarten and Michael, 2009a; Rosengarten and Michael, 2009b). The following statement explains this phenomenon with reference to what may occur within women.

> There could be differences in drug exposure because of genetics, there could be differences in drug exposure because of environment, because of dietary influences, or nutrition or malnutrition issues as well, so different populations could definitely have different exposures. So we have evaluated blood plasma exposures ... but also evaluated exposures in the cervico-vaginal secretions of women. ... Clearly, infection occurs at the mucosal surface, or in that first mucosal layer, so what we've assumed is that the concentration in the tissues is somewhere between the concentration in blood plasma and the concentration in the cervico-vaginal fluid, because the drug has to

> track from the blood – when taken orally – from the blood, through the tissues, and then into the cervico-vaginal fluid .... And what we found is that certain drugs concentrated in the vaginal fluid, compared to blood plasma, are four, five, or six-fold higher in the vaginal fluid than in blood plasma. And other drugs were much lower in the vaginal fluid than in blood plasma – 1 per cent, 10 per cent of what we saw in blood plasma. So the drugs themselves, the physical chemical properties of the drugs themselves, are very different, and produce very different results, depending upon which drug you're looking at.
>
> (R11)

The next quote also discusses PrEP in relation to women but the emphasis is on how PrEP might function in generating new social relations outside the body.

> We're certainly in a situation in which this [PrEP] could be the ultimate female controlled method, because if it doesn't have to be applied genitally, then there shouldn't be any reason that the woman's partner would know that they're doing anything for prevention. It shouldn't in any way interfere with sexual activity, that can still go on in whatever way the couple chooses for that to go on. But for women where they may have ... women in situations in which they don't feel that they have the ability to make open decisions with their partners ... we also want to be careful that it's not exploited in some way. For instance, a study of vaccine attitudes in the Dominican Republic found, when they interviewed sex workers, the female sex workers were excited about vaccine research, but they also said: 'We're concerned that if we find a safe and effective vaccine, that men will use that as a reason to ... to not use condoms, and we won't be able to get them to use condoms, because they'll say, "No, you're going to get the vaccine", or "You've gotten the vaccine, and therefore I refuse to use condoms"'. And what the men said was, 'A vaccine would be great, because then I'll refuse to use condoms', and 'I can have as many partners as I want'. So you wouldn't want there to be a situation like that with PrEP either. I think that we should never assume that any of these strategies is going to be a hundred per cent safe and effective, and I think we're going to still have to find ways to protect women and men from exposures that they don't want to have.
>
> (R04)

The statement is not especially surprising. As we indicated earlier, many HIV scientists are now acutely aware of 'disinhibition'. Importantly, though, it is conceived according to a model of human agency that assumes biotechnologies to be 'good' or 'neutral' but subject to the vagaries of a human capacity to perform them incorrectly (Rosengarten, 2009). Yet when it comes to thinking about 'disinhibition' in relation to women it becomes difficult to sustain this overly simplified account of the work of biotechnological interventions, especially when it is necessary to explain the emergence of unwanted phenomena. PrEP may reduce some women's reliance on a male partner's use of condoms. But it may also affect the thinking and acting of male sexual subjects in a manner that comes to be embodied in women, not dissimilar in some respects to the way women's bodies bear the consequences of hormonal contraception. From this perspective, the use of PrEP could contribute to an already sex differentiated field where higher risk and rates of HIV infection for women are replaced by embodied risk of drug side effects requiring medical surveillance, *actual* drug side effects, demands of dosing adherence and, depending on levels of embodied 'partial effectiveness', continued, even though likely to be reduced, rates of HIV. The relationship between PrEP and women is one example of how PrEP may have multiple functionalities that will emerge in its relations with users and these functionalities may extend beyond what is currently framed as safe and effective HIV prevention to other areas of socio-material life.

Ethics, ontological openness and prevention assemblages

In the remainder of the chapter we concentrate on what an alternative approach might involve, given the dynamic processual nature of PrEP – including its potential gender dimensions – and what might be more usefully understood through the notion of multiple ontologies or ontological openness (Mol, 2003). We begin with a review of two papers focused on HIV biomedical trials that attempt to extend the scope of bioethics and to extract from the experience of the early PrEP trials some lessons for more effective relations between researchers and the researched. We use the arguments put forward in these papers to segue into recent work undertaken outside the HIV field that focuses on a more relational dynamic involving, in the first instance, a methadone clinic (Gomart, 2004) and, secondly, the functionality of the drug Viagra to facilitate multiple conceptions of satisfactory sexual experiences (even when the drug appears not to work) (Potts, 2004). These studies offer an alternative conceptual framework for undertaking further enquiry into HIV biomedical trials including, but not only, PrEP. They demonstrate the potential of working with complexity, moreover, in a manner more compatible with the heterogeneity and multiplicity that can be identified in the current challenge of HIV prevention as the field becomes increasingly affected by biomedicine (Rosengarten, 2009).

In a paper titled 'Enrolling women into HIV preventive vaccine trials: an ethical imperative but a logistical challenge' by Edward Mills et al. (2006), we find one of the few attempts within the HIV literature to review how ethics are enacted in relation to biomedical prevention trials. The paper sets out to highlight a world where female trial volunteers live complex lives that not only *interfere* with the conduct required by the trial (for example, attending regular clinical consultations at a clinic, regular dosing, using contraception), the trial may *interfere* with daily as well as long term *life*. The aim of the paper in making apparent the challenges faced by enrolling women and especially women at high risk of becoming infected with HIV is to ensure that the needs of this group are not ignored. This enables us to gain some sense of what comes to comprise 'a trial' and its aftermath. Although acknowledged as 'basic', they offer a list of requirements to make a trial gender sensitive. These include the siting of a trial in a location convenient to the participants, welcoming reception spaces, privacy for interviews to ensure confidentiality, comfortable and child friendly waiting areas, childcare during examinations, clean toilets, canteen and appropriate audiovisual material and literature on HIV prevention.[10] The list locates scientific testing in a broader network of relations as it considers the contributory work of the everyday. In doing so it contributes – along with the extended relations involved in intercurrent infection to our sense that bioethics premised on only human-to-human relations are insufficient for grasping the relations engendered by a trial. Further it indicates that the everyday is part of the making of a biomedical trial. Ethics are imbued in the trial as the latter functions as a technology for bringing people and drugs together in particular ways.

Although the Mills et al. (2006) paper does not address the critical effects of the biomedical technology, an earlier paper, also lead-authored by Mills, provides another opportunity to foreground the implicit presence of the inter-relationality between otherwise presumed distinct areas of social and material life. Titled 'Designing research in vulnerable populations: lessons from HIV prevention trials that stopped early' (Mills et al., 2005), the paper proposes that consumer research, founded on social marketing principles, could provide a means of tailoring trials to be more inclusive of trial participant interests. The authors note that this strategy has been valuable in the past for shaping the development of effective HIV prevention education (2005: 1404). Either wittingly or unwittingly, such messages have facilitated practices that engage with the virus as more or other than a biological entity. Indeed, when Tony Barnett and Alan Whiteside (2006: 41) contend that, '[f]ortunately for humankind, HIV is not a robust virus and it is hard to transmit', they draw attention to an epidemic that is enabled by more than a mere biological agent. In having a 'social life', its viability is explicitly mediated by the way in which humans engage and are engaged by technologies of knowledge, now including pharmaceutical technologies (Kippax, 2005; Kippax and Race, 2003; Rosengarten, 2009). In other words, despite the enactment by science of the virus as a stable object, its effects reveal it to be already a mix of phenomena beyond simply semiotic (symbolic or cultural) and material (biological) (Haraway, 1991; Treichler, 1999).

In the study undertaken by Emilie Gomart on a methadone substitution clinic for heroin users, the problematic of stable objects is overcome by the adoption of an ethnographic approach designed to allow the emergence of subjects through their relations with the methadone service (2004). Notable is the intentional excluding of a presumption that the clients possess individual agency on the basis of which they could be prejudged or seen to be a slave to or master of the drug, as if client and drug are separate. Gomart states that the aim of her study was to seek out how the drug (methadone) 'performs the user as active and, in turn, is performed through the activity of the user' (2004: 105). Chemical constraints therefore became 'opportunities' for the activity or learning of the user, rather than as more usually deemed: 'obstacles'. Such opportunities provide conditions for devising styles of living that may be found effective by different individuals using or running the clinic. Following Gomart's work, PrEP trials could be seen to provide opportunities to study at close hand – even if in a more determined context than the usual everyday – the performative nature of PrEP trial *design*. For instance in the context of existing trial design, it may be possible to ask: in what ways does PrEP – as it is currently formulated and prescribed – provide embodied opportunities for devising styles of living that do not transmit virus? In this way, bioethics is extended to broader considerations of how trials achieve ethically effective prevention. In instances where prevention practices are increased, as noted with some vaccine trials, it is apparent that the technology of the trial has the potential to be part of the broader goal of prevention and not simply biomedical efficacy (Grant et al., 2005). Or, in line with the emphasis on how technologies bring entities together (Michael, 2006), it may be important to ask in what ways do trial protocols and all their paraphernalia mix human and pharmaceutical? In what ways do consent forms presume and require a mix of social conduct with medicalised conduct on the part of the trial participant? Further, in what ways do the protocols seek to materialise newly abled or disabled bodies, that is, hybridised forms through their enrolment and what distinctions do they draw between trial populations and the broader populations in which the trial is situated.

The above questions constitute a different methodological style that begins from the recognition that the natural and cultural are in a constant state of exchange (Michael, 2006; Rosengarten, 2009). In a recent account of the drug Viagra by Annie Potts we are reminded of the many possibilities that may emerge in an exchange specifically involving a body–drug relation. Consistent with Gomart's argument that excludes a prior concept of human agency, for Potts there is no prior given body. There are only [ever] bodies that are 'created through temporary assemblages that may involve connections between the organic and inorganic' (2004: 19). This means that bodies, to quote Potts: 'must not be interpreted according to their meanings or identities, but rather with reference to what they do.' We could apply this approach to PrEP trial participants and claim that they are not simply 'trail participants' asked to test a drug and on the basis of which test results can be generalised to others presumed to be represented by the participants. Rather, trial participants emerge as part of an assemblage inclusive of the trial design, historically engendered local specificities, drug effects, potential exposure to virus, possible engagement in risk practices, possible HIV infection and partner or partners who may be HIV positive. This mix means that the assemblage is always in process and the entities that comprise it are altering of each other (Potts, 2004: 22; Gomart, 2004; Mol and Law, 2004: 45). Following the style of questioning we proposed above and derived from Gomart and Potts' work, here we might ask: what can a PrEP assemblage do? What set of associations involving drugs and bodies acts with or against safe and effective prevention? Or, to take a step back from the focus on bodies and drugs, we could ask: how do trials give the appearance of one set of associations in play while performing others? In what way might prevention benefit by excluding human agency or extending agency across the terrain of associations? Any of these questions, if pursued, will help perform an alternative conception of prevention. Most specifically, they underscore how prevention is ontologically open and, most importantly, in the sense that what is conceived and enacted as prevention can be altered.

Conclusion

> It's hard to imagine who it [PrEP] will be targeted to, and for how long.
>
> (R20)

As we have shown, the question of who PrEP may be suitable for is not anticipated to be answered in full by the results of current trials. While these may achieve a level of conceptual stability through established and highly sophisticated modes of statistical standardisation, they will not necessarily enable the achievement of safe and effective prevention. Nor will recourse to lessons drawn from prior experience of non-biomedical prevention and from the experience of treatment and its effects on 'disinhibition' necessarily be 'successful', although we do not deny this too will be valuable. The voices of early opposition to the trials, the work of Mills et al. (2006) and, indeed, Grant et al. (2005) all, in their own way, indicate that the functionality of PrEP will be processual, involving the continuing relational workings of 'biological' and 'social' phenomena. Determining those for whom PrEP will be suitable will be contingent on how this dynamic relationality is enabled to emerge. Putting this another way, the value of PrEP is woven into the very composition of the PrEP assemblage in its developing specificity. Therefore, PrEP also serves as an example of how HIV prevention more generally is an assemblage: in this instance it is composed of drugs but, inevitably, of bodies, knowledges or lack thereof, assumptions, styles of engagement and virus in a serodiscordant human-to-human relation involving routes of transmission. Safe and effective prevention will require a capacity to conceptualise the context-specific processual of the assemblage – biomedical and otherwise – and to access the open systems that such assemblages mediate. A corollary step is to consider how particular relations within the assemblage can be relatively strengthened or weakened, commissioned or decommissioned. However this pans out in particular cases, the very conceptualisation in terms of assemblage alerts us to the fact that this will always be a process fraught with complex ramifications and unintended consequences.

Acknowledgements

In addition to the two anonymous referees and the editors, we are grateful to Mitchell Warren, AIDS Vaccine Advocacy Coalition (AVAC) and Dean

Murphy, previously Australian Federation of AIDS Organisations (AFAO), who assisted with relevant literature and access to key stakeholders in PrEP. We would also like to acknowledge the support provided by Goldsmiths Research and Knowledge Transfer Fund and the Foundation for the Sociology of Health and Illness.

References

AVAC (AIDS Vaccine Advocacy Coalition) (2005) *Will a Pill a Day Prevent HIV? Anticipating the Results of PREP Trials* (New York: AVAC).

—— (2008) *Anticipating the Results of PrEP Trials* (New York: AVAC).

Barnett, T. and Whiteside, A. (2006) *AIDS in the Twenty-First Century: Disease and Globalization* (second ed.) (Basingstoke, UK: Palgrave Macmillan).

Bass, E. & Kahn, P. (2005) 'Testing AIDS Vaccines in People' *AIDS Vaccine Handbook: Global Perspectives* (second ed.) (ed.) Patricia Kahn (New York: AIDS Vaccine Advocacy Coalition).

Gomart, E. (2004) 'Surprised by Methadone: In Praise of Drug Substitution Treatment in a French Clinic', *Body & Society*, 10 (2–3): 85–110.

Grant, R. M., Buchbinder, S., Cates, W., Clarke, E., Coates, T., Cohen, M. S., Delaney, M., Flores, G., Goicochea, P., Gonsalves, G., Harrington, M., Lama, J. R., MacQueen, K. M., Moore, J. P., Peterson, L., Sanchez, J., Thompson, M., Wainberg, M. A. (2005) 'AIDS: Promote HIV Chemoprophylaxis Research, Don't Prevent It', *Science*, 30, September: 2170–1.

Haraway, D. (1991) *Simians, Cyborgs, and Women: The Reinvention of Nature* (London: Free Association Books).

Jintarkanon, S., Nakapiew, S., Tienudom, N., Suwannawong, P. and Wilson, D. (2005) 'Unethical Clinical Trials in Thailand: A Community Response', *Lancet*, 365: 1617–18.

Kippax, S. (2005) 'Pre-Exposure Prophylaxis (PREP)', PREP Forum, Cockle Bay, Australia, 16 June.

Kippax, S., and K. Race (2003) 'Sustaining Safe Practice: Twenty Years On', *Social Science & Medicine*, 57: 1–12.

MacQueen, K. M., Namey, E., Chilongozi, D. A., Mtweve, S. P., Mlingo, M., Morar, N., Reid, C., Ristow, A., Sahay, S., HPTN 035 Standard Of Care Assessment Team (2007) 'Community Perspectives on Care Options for HIV Prevention Trial Participants', *AIDS Care*, 19 (4): 554–60.

Michael, M. (2006) *Technoscience and Everyday Life: The Complex Simplicities of the Mundane* (UK: Open University Press).

Mills, E., Rachlis, B., Wu, P., Wong, E., Wilson, K. and Singh, S. (2005) 'Media Reporting of Tenofovir Trials in Cambodia and Cameroon', *BMC International Health and Human Rights*, 5 (6): 1–7.

Mills, E., Nixon, S., Singh, S., Dolma, S., Nayyar, A. and Kapoor, S. (2006) 'Enrolling Women into HIV Preventive Vaccine Trials: An Ethical Imperative but a Logistical Challenge', *PLoS Medicine*, March, 3 (3, e94): 1–4.

Mol, A. (2003) *The Body Multiple: Ontology in Medical Practice* (Durham: Duke University Press).

Mol, A. and Law, J. (2004) 'Embodied Action, Enacted Bodies: The example of Hypoglycaemia', *Body & Society*, 10 (2–3): 43–62.

Page-Shafer, K., Saphonn, V., Penh Sun, L., Chhi Vun, M., Cooper, D. A. and Kaldor, J. M. (2005) 'HIV Prevention Research in a Resource-limited Setting: The Experience of Planning a Trial in Cambodia', *The Lancet*, 366: 1499–503.

Paxton, L. A., Hope, T. and Jaffe, H. W. (2007) 'Pre-exposure Prophylaxis for HIV Infection: What if it works?', *Lancet*, 370: 89–93.

Potts, A. (2004) 'Deleuze on Viagra (Or, What Can a 'Viagra-body' Do?)', *Body & Society*, 10 (1): 17–36.

Rosengarten, M. (2009) *HIV Interventions: Biomedicine and the Traffic in Information and Flesh* (Seattle/London: University of Washington Press).

Rosengarten, M. and Michael, M. (2009a) 'Rethinking the Bioethical Enactment of Drugged Bodies: On the Paradoxes of using anti-HIV Drug Therapy as a Technology for Prevention', Special Issue on 'Drugged Bodies', *Science as Culture*, Guest editors: Suzanne Fraser, Celia Roberts and Kylie Valentine, 18 (2): 183–99.

—— (2009b) 'The performative function of expectations in translating treatment to prevention: the case of HIV pre-exposure prophylaxis or PrEP', *Social Science and Medicine*, 69 (7): 1049–55.

Singh, J. A. and Mills, E. J. (2005) 'The Abandoned Trials of Pre-Exposure Prophylaxis for HIV: What Went Wrong?', *PLoS Medicine*, 2 (9, e234): 0001–4.

The Thai AIDS Treatment Action Group TTATAG (2004) Letter 8 December, available at: http://www.aidsinfonyc.org/tag/activism/thaiTenofovir.html.

Treichler, P. (1999) *How to Have Theory in an Epidemic: Cultural Chronicles of AIDS* (Durham, NC: Duke University Press).

WHO/UNAIDS (2004) 'Treating People with Intercurrent Infection in HIV Prevention Trials, Report from a WHO/UNAIDS consultation, Geneva 17–18 July 2003 p. 1', *AIDS*, 21 (18, 15): W1–12.

UNAIDS/WHO (2007) Press Release. Available at: http://data.unaids.org/pub/EPISlides/2007/071119_epi_pressrelease_en.pdf.

Venn, C. (2006) 'A Note on Assemblage', *Theory, Culture & Society*, 23, (2–3): 107–8.

Notes

1. The brand name for Tenofovir is Viread® or Tenofovir Disoproxil Fumarate. The brand name is Viread® (or Tenofovir Disoproxil Fumarate) and the brand name is Emtriva®.
2. MTCP or mother-to-child prevention of HIV transmission is an internationally condoned strategy to prevent HIV transmission. Risk of prevention is reduced to under two per cent by the inclusion of antiretroviral drugs during pregnancy and labour to the infant in the first weeks of life, plus complete avoidance of breastfeeding. See http://www.who.int/hiv/pub/guidelines/pmtct/en/index.html. It is difficult to establish the effectiveness of PEP in non-occupational exposures as it is very difficult to confirm that exposure has already taken place. However, the evidence from MTCP and from its use in occupational exposures has led to the development of international guidelines for its usage. See 'Post Exposure Prophylaxis Following Non-Occupational Exposures' Background Document Prepared by Michelle Roland, University of California, San Francisco, for the Joint ILO/WHO Technical Meeting for the Development of Guidelines and Policies on

Occupational and Non-Occupational Post Exposure Prophylaxis (PEP), Geneva, 2005.

3. For a full list of trials in operation and planned, see http://www.prepwatch.org/trials.htm.
4. The trials have been initiated by independent teams of researchers and are sponsored by the US National Institute of Allergy and Infectious Diseases (NIAID), the US Centers for Disease Control and Prevention (CDC) and Family Health International (FHI) with funding from the Bill and Melinda Gates Foundation.
5. Mills et al. (2005) 'Designing research in vulnerable populations: lessons from HIV prevention trials that stopped early' *BMJ*, 331: 1403–6.
6. It has not been possible to find a documented explanation of the final decision by Family Health International. Anecdotal reporting suggests that it was no longer possible to continue the trial after such a break.
7. The Cambodian study was funded by the NIAID, part of the US National Institutes of Health, and by the University of New South Wales with funding administered by Family Health International. On final approval the funding was to be administered by NIAID. The study was planned and intended to be conducted by the Cambodian National Centre for HIV, AIDS, Dermatology and STDs (NCHADS), Phnom Penh, Cambodia; the University of California San Francisco (UCSF) and the University of New South Wales (UNSW), Sydney, Australia. It may be important to mention that both were aided by the French group 'Paris Act Up'.
8. In some instances oversight committees are termed 'Institutional Review Boards' or 'Independent Data Monitoring Committees'.
9. As one of our interviewees stated: 'We train local people in everything which has to do with the trial, and one can transfer that to many other capacities. We go over everything like we ask local people how to counsel the participants, everybody who will be a counsellor in the trial is trained on the standard of how do you counsel risk reduction for women, how do you counsel contraceptive use, how do you enter data in a database, how do you verify that your entry is correct, how do you do all the lab procedures – how do you document a sample, how do you treat a sample' (R05).
10. Mills, E., Nixon, S., Singh, S., Dolma, S., Nayyar, A. and Kapoor, S. (2006) 'Enrolling women into HIV preventive vaccine trials: an ethical imperative but a logistical challenge' in *PLoS Medicine*, March, 3 (3, e94), 1–4, p. 0310.

10
Particularity, Potentiation, Citizenship and Pragmatism

Mark Davis and Corinne Squire

Introduction

The case studies presented in this volume have addressed HIV technologies as formations of the material, embodied, social and political in modes of engagement with the HIV epidemic. As argued throughout, this notion of HIV technologies is needed to grapple with the particularities of the HIV pandemic in the treatment possibility era. This approach provides a way of conceptualising HIV medical, social, cultural and political treatment and prevention technologies and their hybrids. The perspective draws attention to the sociocultural and political aspects of HIV medical treatment technologies and to the increasingly biotechnical bases for HIV prevention. It also encourages reflection on forms of HIV prevention and social care that are not typically understood as technologies but that, as has been demonstrated, share many structural and political features with technical, biomedical means of addressing HIV. This perspective can also allow us to grapple with relations between treatment and prevention, as many of the chapters in this volume have demonstrated.

Adopting this general approach and extending it in innovative ways, each of the chapters have addressed the familiar and important HIV technologies that inform national and international efforts to address the HIV epidemic. Campbell has explored and critiqued community participation in HIV interventions in sub-Saharan Africa. Abdullah and Squire have identified the salience of locally democratic partnership in implementing HIV treatment in resource-constrained settings in South Africa. Mykhalovskiy analysed the history, benefits and drawbacks of the move to integrate HIV treatment and prevention in Canada. By drawing on qualitative interview data and group discussion, other chapters have considered intersubjective HIV technologies. Wilbraham considered the psychosocial dimensions of South African print media encouraging parental care about the sexual health of children. In UK settings, Flowers explored the transitions in living with HIV that are necessary in the era of access to ART, and Davis examined the ethical implications of the knowledge produced in and around the effects of ART on the risk of HIV transmission in sexual practice. Other chapters in this volume have considered some of the effects of biomedical technologies of HIV prevention. With reference to the use of HIV antibody blood testing to ascertain serostatus, Race examined discourse concerning unsafe sex among gay men and in particular barebacking in developed world contexts. Rosengarten and Michael developed the notion of transnational clinical trials for pre-exposure prophylaxis (PrEP) as both problematic and productive sites for HIV prevention activity.

These critical studies of HIV technologies have sought to question prevailing assumptions regarding the apparent technologisation, and specifically biomedicalisation, of approaches to the HIV epidemic. The studies have also expanded definitions of HIV technologies, and questioned the technologies themselves, thus enabling new modes of critical understanding and analysis. In this concluding chapter, we would like to draw attention to four main cross-cutting themes from the case studies: particularity, played out in chapters' carefully specified and interrelated concerns; potentiation, understood here as the technical, ethical and political interrelations through which the effects of HIV technologies can change; tensions in the kinds of HIV citizenship associated with HIV technologies; and the pragmatics or 'practical truths' that are being negotiated in and around the everyday use of HIV technologies and how such practices and insights themselves serve as counterpoints to more distanced, generalised and uncontested efforts to govern via HIV technologies.

Particularity

A central endeavour in this project has been to sustain depictions that pay attention to the particular conditions and expressions of the HIV epidemic in trans- and intra-national contexts. Neglecting such particularities, even when they cannot be fully specified and addressed, is recognised as a shortfall in engagements with the pandemic (Campbell, 2003). We suggest that recognising particularity is also a necessary precondition for HIV activists and advocators, service providers, policy-makers and theoreticians, if they are to articulate and act on relations and alliances between those particularities (Laclau and Mouffe, 2001 [1985]). This volume moves beyond globalising dichotomies and reductive analyses towards situated accounts of HIV technologies and their ramifications which recognise their multipolar attachments and investments (Mouffe; 2005). The volume's notion of HIV technologies as complex assemblages embracing both HIV treatment and prevention, biomedical and sociocultural formations, and physical, social and symbolic resources is useful because it draws all these fields into articulations of particularity. In the process, it helps resist some of the dichotomies that are common in the HIV field and beyond. Chapters in this volume have exploded 'developed versus developing' country discourse, questioned simple notions of before and after the advent of ART and challenged reductive approaches to the tension between human agency and biomedical power. They have addressed the HIV pandemic's divergent historical moments, paying attention to the specific histories of HIV epidemics across varying global locations, nation states and intra-national social groups. Particularity is also worked out through the volume's address to the 'psychosocial', most clearly in Flowers's emphasis on the neglect of psychosocial engagements with HIV epidemics. Chapter writers have also traced the related and autonomous operations of biomedical and sociocultural HIV technologies in their particular socio-temporal contexts of production, translation and application. Rosengarten and Michael's exploration of the biomedical and sociopolitical technological assemblages surrounding PrEP exemplifies this thoroughgoing engagement with the particularities of HIV technologies.

The volume has also worked across different methodological approaches, addressing HIV technologies via the heterogeneous set of epistemological positions which can articulate them. It has included case studies derived from large-scale HIV interventions, analyses of research and policy from different country contexts, historical perspectives on HIV technologies and close focus qualitative research with people affected by HIV. For example, Campbell provided a meta-analysis of evaluations of HIV education and care programmes in South Africa and Zimbabwe up to the early 2000s – in many of which she was herself involved – programmes that remain salient for the situations of uneven treatment and care that still characterise most high HIV prevalence nations. Abdullah and Squire drew predominantly on the documentation and ethnography of policy, to show how particularity in the contemporary HIV era has to do with the mixing of universal treatment possibility with uneven provision and resources.

The chapters in this volume also consistently address the multipolar power relations in HIV technologies. Writers' address to 'community' is an obvious example. Campbell, Abdullah and Squire, and Mykhalovskiy, for instance, analyse the difficult term 'community' in distinct contexts of technological hierarchy and negotiation, and come to specific conclusions: respectively, that 'community' is simultaneously invoked and erased by HIV programmes; that 'community' can have a contingent but important effect on those programmes, given certain 'partnership' technologies; and that 'community' is always positioned in opposition to other forces and has repeatedly to be re-inscribed. These findings, while particular to each of the chapters' investigatory contexts, have some generality of application outside those contexts, and they are commensurable with each other. All three chapters position 'community' as a complicated and problematic term that can still have something to offer for people's collective organisation and action 'technologies' around HIV.

Similarly, Wilbraham positions the politics of South African HIV prevention as nationally specific, but also transnational, and suggests that difficulties in addressing such complexity leads to prevention discourses' limited effectivity. Drawing on her own group interviews, she argues that interviewees discursively adopt the value 'talking to children about sex' as part of a 'sexual citizenship' at least partly translated from western, white, middle class discourse, involving open talk about feelings, rights and responsibilities. However, this talk is also, she suggests, part of a South Africa-specific commitment to engage with problems around family life and the HIV epidemic, and a manifestation of South African discourses of the sociality of childhood, and of classed urban progress, cultural change, and emergence from apartheid-mandated ignorance.

A further particularity related to HIV technologies pertains to contemporary social theory. For example, it is not easy to reconcile the specificities discussed here with the canonic critique of the neoliberal individualisation of modern systems of health care. Plainly such critiques are not sufficient, as this volume indicates. Not all HIV contexts are individualising, and within contemporary HIV governance lies a great variety of technologies of autonomy and self-subjection. A straightforward critique of neoliberalisation of and through HIV technologies is too totalising for the transnational yet fine-grained perspectives provided here. Moreover, some discourses of HIV technologies' possibility and contingency reveal surprising turnings and unexpected lacunae that do not fit well with simple theoretical accounts of their productive or resistant, progressive or conservative nature. Chapters in this volume underline such particularities and point us towards methods of analysis that can take account of them. For example, Race and Rosengarten and Michael revealed both the problematic and productive aspects of HIV technologies. Race showed that elements of the practice of barebacking are enormously productive forms of agentic engagement with biomedical technologies, such as the HIV antibody blood test and ART, and do not necessarily lead to HIV transmission. Race acknowledged that such developments are not without problems but suggested that the interrogation of these is clouded by pre-emptive accounts of changes in sexual practice and related interventions. These conflicted opportunities and challenges in HIV technologies appear in relation to the HIV virus itself. Rosengarten and Michael have shown how the persistence of assumptions of a notional HIV as a stable biological singularity misses out on how its 'viability', as they refer to it, depends on society, culture and selves.

A commitment to understanding particularity directs us to the least noticeable and most ignored aspects of the interrelated and multipolar relations of power at play in the pandemic. At the same time, such analysis has to negotiate particularity with comprehensibility, persuasiveness and political feasibility. As Race (this volume) argues, particularity is inevitable when addressing the multiple-lived technologies of the epidemic, but it is at the same time necessary to compromise such particularity in order to find terms of engagement. A cross-cutting component of these requirements is the analysis of directions within particularity that connect HIV technologies across fields and across time, and that extrapolate into spatial and temporal futures, engendering technological breaks and shifts in the process. Such an analysis moves away from particularity towards what we are calling technological potentiation.

Potentiation

The common meaning of potentiation is 'transfer of power'. This initial meaning is one way and electrical, but technologies can of course metaphorically potentiate each other; and power, taking many forms, can work in different directions (Foucault, 1980), turning the well-predicted changes of electrical potentiation into moves towards possibilities. We can also understand potentiation as an instantiation of Deleuze's account of the virtual which he distinguishes from the possible (Deleuze and Parnet, 1977) in respect of the lack of relation between its ground and its actualisation: what is to come is not predictable, does not inhere in what is already with us, but this future is nonetheless seeded by the processes, rather than the contents, of the present. Potentiation concretises the move from virtual to real by specifying the different objects, states or phenomena from whose relation the virtual comes into reality, by acknowledging the shifts in power that produce that change and by predicting, necessarily imperfectly, directions of change. In these processes, potentiation in fact comes close to Laclau and Mouffe's (1985) notion of hegemonic articulations, built up from particularities towards a universality that is always contingent and contested. From exchange and contest between HIV technologies, derive different technologies – not necessarily better, but offering other routes towards living with and understanding HIV.

Countries living long-term with high-prevalence HIV epidemics are clearly going to undergo potentiations across HIV technologies of diagnosis, treatment, care and education, and in interaction with the other difficult technologies of lives lived in resource-constrained circumstances, of kinds that cannot easily be predicted over the next few decades. Magona (2008) suggests in the South African context that for women, the potentiation of technologies of sexual and other self-determinations may be one result of long-term living with the virus. Another result may be the normalising of HIV, though in a different way to that remarked in the developed world. In high-prevalence contexts this often seems to be happening through discourses of 'AIDS fatigue', articulated by the HIV infected, affected and unaffected alike, and through small-scale but indicative practices like the use of male and female condoms as footballs, toys and jewellery. HIV-associated objects are multifunctional resources in resource-poor contexts, as well as objects with powerful meanings that might be defused by these diverse functions. Such social normalisation will no doubt always, as in developed-world biomedical normalisation, be haunted by its obverse; displayed for instance in the increasing representational separation off of 'the HIV positive', who are often also marked by gender and poverty (Lana, 2009; Steinberg, 2008). This move is in turn strongly resisted by some political and media articulations like, in South Africa, the *Sowetan* newspaper column written by Lucky Mazibuko (2008), repeatedly reminding his readers over the last ten years that HIV positive people cannot be secreted away.

How does the potentiation of HIV technologies play out in this book? We have seen throughout that lines of potential change may be constructed and then extrapolated from analyses of particularity. Wilbraham, for example, suggests working across the limits of prevention technologies that she delimits to imagine other technologies. Moving between historical moments in the relation between technologies of HIV prevention and treatment, Mykhalovskiy suggests the possibility of reconfiguring 'responsibility', from the perspective of everyday HIV lives and activism. All the writers who address 'community' look across the fractures within this field, towards potential other futures.

A powerful example of potentiation comes from writers' formulations of connections between prevention and treatment technologies. Derived from their commitment to analysing particularity and multipolarity, the book chapters support the view that HIV treatment and prevention are mutually potentiating. Such mutual influence is part of many forms and levels of HIV discourse. The clinical effects of ART are said to contribute to prevention, and HIV education is claimed by local HIV organisations and international NGOs alike to assist treatment outcomes, for instance. Potentiation also occurs physiologically in the synergistic effects of various drug combinations. ART itself comprises substances that potentiate one another in the sense that they act on viral replication in different multiplicative ways to therefore reduce or halt it. This volume shows that the concept of potentiation can also be used to draw attention to the social practices that are part of HIV technologies. The argument of the book has been that unless the potentiations between social and biomedical technologies, and between social technologies themselves, are adequately addressed, it will not be possible to achieve planned and hoped-for effects on mortality, morbidity and HIV transmission.

Potentiation permits ways of thinking about the ART era as a mix of technological effects extending from the virus itself, to new languages of possibility and risk, and new modes of governance and self-regulation. The ART era is often typified as marked by a biomedical watershed: the advent of effective HIV treatment. It has been the argument in these chapters that the advent of ART is not a singular break in the history of the pandemic. Junctures and disjunctures abound in this history, alongside reconfigurations of existing, dynamic assemblages of HIV technologies, including those that address the treatment of HIV. In this view, the idea of technological 'watershed' is one way of reflecting on HIV technologies in time, and finding and deliberating on new and useful formations of HIV technologies. 'Techno-watershed' can be therefore taken to express Rabinow's conceptualisation of biosociality intersecting with, and helping to constitute, the history of the HIV epidemic and the technologisation of its governance (Rabinow, 1999). Moreover, such engagements with technologies in time allows the conduct, in everyday lives, the practices of social welfare, large-scale policymaking and academic theory alike, of something analogous to Rabinow's 'anthropology of the contemporary' which enables an address to the question of 'how older and newer elements are given form and worked together' (2007: 2–3).

This concept of biosocial potentiation also addresses some of the problems of dichotomising, 'for' or 'against' approaches to biomedical treatment and prevention technologies. For example, Abdullah and Squire have argued that the effectiveness of ART in South Africa's Western Cape is partly reliant on the social processes that previously sustained prevention, care and some earlier treatment activities. Local, disseminated provision of ART in primary care settings depends strongly on active alliances with interested community-based organisations. This argument suggests that it is not treatment and prevention per se that potentiate each other, but rather the actions of communities of interest and the agencies that support them.

An analysis of potentiation also addresses the common assertion that ART will displace or downgrade prevention activity. This notion is heterogeneous, articulated largely as a matter of shifts in risk perception and practice and governance failure in the developed world, and as capacity failure in the developing world. Abdullah and Squire argued that in the case of the Western Cape, where much attention has been devoted to developing effective partnerships and a community-based ART strategy, the tension between treatment and prevention was less pronounced, despite resource constraints, because the same practitioners and lay actors were involved in both HIV prevention and ART provision. Moreover, in high-prevalence, high-incidence, low-resourced contexts, treatment and prevention present themselves as joint imperatives more forcefully and ubiquitously – though not necessarily more effectively – than in lower-prevalence, well-resourced situations. This argument implies that relations or non-relations between treatment and prevention are not ontological, but discursive, attributable to the prevailing organisational structures and epidemiological contexts of treatment and prevention technologies.

Controversy surrounding the effects of ART on prevention in contexts where treatment is generally available, predominantly in the developed world, also illustrates the value of the concept of potentiation. Typically, debates have circulated around how ART might reconfigure or disrupt HIV prevention and then by reversal, how ART can be applied to meet HIV prevention goals. This simple conceptualisation of ART and prevention inter-determination misses the potentiating aspects of the relationship, and its resonances for related biomedical and social technologies. Perhaps the best-known instantiation of this limited view is the notion of disinhibition, discussed in several chapters in this volume. As is well known, at around the time of its introduction in developed country contexts, researchers began to consider if ART was leading to the reduction of the use of condoms in sexual intercourse (Dilley et al., 1997; Kelly et al., 1998) and made links between such practices and HIV antibody serostatus (Remien et al. 1998). As Rosengarten and Michael noted, the concept of ART's disinhibiting effects has been used to conceptualise these developments. But as has also been shown repeatedly, it is not easy to attribute changes in sexual practice to the advent of ART (Elford, 2006). There are also instructive countervailing applications of the disinhibition thesis. Davis noted how disinhibition, or 'treatment optimism' in his analysis, is seen by some to undermine safer sex among gay men, creating questions over the ethical use of knowledge derived from the clinical management of HIV infection. Rosengarten and Michael showed how disinhibition has been used to argue against trials of PrEP. The disinhibition thesis can thus be used to justify closer attention to the ethical qualities of the sexual practices of those using ART but also as a basis for arguments concerning the possible unethical dimensions of biotechnological methods of HIV prevention and the research methods being used to develop them. These multiple uses of the conceptual framework of disinhibition and the putative effects of ART and related knowledge are significant clues to the particularities in the potentiation of ART and HIV prevention. Knowledge and ethics are at stake in the disinhibition thesis, but with multiple applications and effects in the administration of the HIV epidemic. As Rosengarten and Michael pointed out, to engage with this situation we need to accept the 'dynamic processual nature' of HIV technologies, their social, cultural and political dimensions, and especially their multipolar ethical formations, as the example of disinhibition suggests.

Also addressing the potentiation of HIV prevention and treatment technologies, Mykhalovskiy's chapter suggested that the anxiety about the impact of ART on HIV prevention is not the only relationship that has salience in the treatment possibility era and that there is good reason to address how HIV prevention is reconfiguring the practice of HIV treatment. Mykhalovskiy considered how, in the ART possibility era, the Canadian AIDS Treatment Information Exchange, a community-based treatment advocacy agency, shifted its focus from HIV treatment advocacy, becoming a national agency addressing HIV through a discourse of treatment and prevention integration. Mykhalovskiy argued that in the integration era, the epidemiological rationality of disease control and its language of transmission vectors are sometimes used to help frame the use of ART by people with HIV. ART, ostensibly a treatment for infection, and a hard-won one at that, is now understood by some as a means of preventing HIV transmission. Mykhalovskiy argued that before the development of effective treatment, biomedical HIV technologies were neglected by policymakers and often criticised by activists focused on social technologies of prevention and care. Later, during the biomedical development of ART, the treatment needs of people living with HIV continued to be neglected within medical and social technologies, but were strongly articulated by activists. In the ART possibility era, the medical, social and, to some extent, activist focus has turned to anxiety that people with HIV might not use biomedical technologies properly, often referred to as the problem of adherence or compliance. Through contact with epidemiological rationalities, adherence acquires the additional meaning of being a requirement – alongside minimising transmission risk in sexual and drug-using practices – for avoiding HIV transmission.

Similarly, Flowers argued that the biotechnological fix implied by ART has attractions because it promises control of the virus and freedom from the messiness and contingency of psychosocial aspects of living with HIV such as affect, relationships, sexual mores and cultural practice. One aspect of this biotechnical fix is biomedical 'normalisation', for example, the assumptions that HIV antibody testing should be routine and regular because ART has made HIV positive diagnosis into a social status that is not deeply problematic. As Flowers showed in detail, the normalisation of HIV antibody testing is predicated on biologism and a narrow conceptualisation of what it means to have HIV infection. HIV antibody testing contributes to normalisation because it provides the quantitative data for calculating prevalence and incidence, the central practice of epidemiology in general. As Flowers argued, and notwithstanding the importance of testing's relationship to good health practices, including but not restricted to ART, the HIV antibody test remains the source of significant psychosocial status change. But it seems for many that technologies of blood testing and ART are 'proof' that a biological utilitarianism should underpin attempts to prevent HIV.

Combining the arguments of Rosengarten and Michael, Mykhalovskiy with that of Flowers, we can see that in the ART possibilities era, epidemiological rationalisation of the relationships between ART and HIV prevention could be said to disembed the HIV subject in the sense that it works to sever the link between the psychosocial aspects of HIV and the experience of HIV infection and its management. Some figurations of HIV technologies insist that the HIV virus is, potentially, under biological control (Davis, 2007). The psychosocial thus becomes extra-HIV, relegated to an idiopathic concern.

The question of HIV subjectivity appeared in other chapters that considered personal experience narratives. Davis showed that self-care among people with HIV is figured as challenging and beneficial, but most importantly as a personalised enterprise, best done when both AIDS and self-care labour are hidden. This approach to HIV care may reinforce the biological reductionism of ART-era normalisation. Such invisibilised and individualised HIV self-technologies appear also in developing world ART contexts (Steinberg, 2008) operating under the pressure of HIV's stigmatisation (Flowers, this volume and Flowers et al., 2006) as much as biomedical normalisation – a phenomenon that suggests the dual action of normalising and stigmatising discourses. However, these processes stand in contrast to the Western Cape example noted by Abdullah and Squire, where, as in other settings (for example, Farmer, 2001), treatment support initiatives are recognised as community-wide, public and constituting everyone as to some degree HIV subjects and citizens. In these contexts, no absolute divide separates subjects from citizens, or the seropositive from those of other statuses. Again, these perspectives alert us to the trans- and intra-national particularities of the ART possibility era.

Citizenship

HIV technologies do not just exist in multipolar and particular formations that change and develop through potentiation. They are also part of larger articulations of contested technologies within broader structures of citizenship. All social relations are traversed by citizenship which is not just a matter of legal status in a locality or nation or world, but of a network of power relations that cross and depart from, reinforce and contradict each other (Mouffe, 1992). Pulled into social existence by these relations, citizens are also inherently ethical beings, provoked into subjecthood by the requirement to situate oneself morally within a range of different fields (Butler, 2005). HIV technologies of all kinds – biomedical, social and cultural – are themselves morally positioned by their citizenly affiliations and are engaged in contests between the different kinds of citizenship that claim and derive from them.

It is notable both how plastic citizenship can be, and how thoroughly imbricated it is with HIV technologies. This embedded significance suggests that citizenship can be taken to be both a presiding principle and an effect of HIV technologies. Because it draws together notions of autonomy and constraint and ethical tensions surrounding social and sexual relations, citizenship can be taken to be the prime governmental site of HIV technologies. It can assist in making HIV technologies work effectively, as in the roll-out of ART in the Western Cape, and it can be a site for the exercise of disciplinary requirements on citizens, as in the case of parent-oriented sex education, considered by Wilbraham. HIV citizenship is unavoidably subject to tension and contestation; flux and contradictions are axiomatic to critical understandings of it.

Citizenship's place in HIV technologies is sometimes manifested in obvious ways – for instance, within Europe, in the conflation of legal arguments about 'reckless' transmission or transmission risk, with political arguments about the citizenship status of migrants, in a number of cases (Monk, 2009). As Race points out (this volume), prevention technologies earlier in the pandemic focused on responsibilising every citizen, not making prevention the responsibility specifically of HIV positive or possibly HIV positive people. Within this dispensation, we were all to some degree HIV citizens. Recent feminised and racialised prosecutions indicate the degree to which developed-world prevention technologies now operate with differentiated citizens, exiled progressively from full citizenship by actual or possible HIV positivity, femininity and migrant or illegal status. Conversely, HIV citizenship technologies still work inclusively in some high-prevalence contexts, at least within policy and activist discourse, setting up zones of equivalence (Mouffe, 1992) between people who are HIV positive and everyone else, since all are to some extent 'living with' the virus, though in different and particular ways. HIV citizenship technologies may also articulate HIV citizenship with other citizenships, as shown by for instance the expansion of Treatment Action Campaign initiatives, from HIV treatment activism towards addressing gender-based violence and xenophobic protests and attacks in South Africa.

As in the last example, the fields of citizenship technologies surrounding HIV break up putative characterisations of such citizenship as monolithically biomedical. Race has shown that safer sex, a sociomedical technology that addresses the prevention of HIV transmission, is also a political and cultural intervention in the HIV epidemic, attributable to the actions of HIV positive and HIV affected citizens. While addressing HIV, safer sex also addresses the ethical basis for sexual relationality and claims on autonomy in the face of a life-threatening epidemic. For this reason, controversy over so-called barebacking, and related debates regarding the use of HIV antibody status to make decisions about whether or not to use condoms for sexual intercourse, need to be seen as reconfigurations of the safer sex technology under pressure from HIV prevention imperatives. As Race demonstrated, barebacking can be understood as a formation of safer sex in the sense that it is a technology of citizenly ethics and care, with a level of psychosocial reflexivity that canonic forms of safer sex may not attain (Fleet, 2009).

Along with such case studies of HIV technologies and their subjects, citizenship emerged in the book as an important framing concept for treatment and prevention programmes. Abdullah and Squire asserted that the specific configurations of HIV treatment citizenship in the Western Cape, connected to histories of political action and the long-lived cultural politics of *ubuntu*, or collective human responsibility, as well as to contemporary and local social-political associations, enabled successful ART roll-out. 'Citizenship' is not by itself an answer, however. Wilbraham examined HIV prevention technologies in South Africa to explore how these 'require and fabricate' (this volume, page 85) forms of HIV citizenship that have clear limits in relation to HIV prevention. Citizenship's variability here works against itself: in its sexualised and individualised form it contests a citizenship of parental, particularly maternal, responsibility which reveals its contingency. Mykhalovskiy's chapter recapitulated citizenly contest, between responsibilised and individualised subjects of HIV technologies. In Davis's chapter, such contests were potentiating: bioinformational citizenship and self-care appeared as technologies of hope that can be effective despite their personalised and secreted characters. This chapter suggested that HIV's bioinformational citizenship needs to be seen biosocially and more broadly, that the sexual citizenship of rational individuals must be reformulated within the frame of informational biocitizenship and the ethics of uncertainty (Rabinow, 2004).

Two chapters addressed HIV technologies' relations with citizenship in informatively transnational frames. Campbell's chapter examined technologies of 'community participation' and 'empowerment' that underpin many programmes funded by international aid agencies in southern Africa. Campbell argued that, far from encouraging forms of HIV citizenship that can moderate the effects of the HIV epidemic and promote risk reduction and social care, these programmes extend power inequalities and perpetuate ineffective interventions. She revealed how community participation and capacity building can defeat itself. What makes HIV programmes effective is known and includes such factors as social spaces for dialogue and critical thinking, shared purpose, acknowledgement of local capacities, and 'bridging capital' which supports effective relationships between local individuals and communities and external and international development agencies. As Campbell showed, many programmes are disappointing because they are poorly administered, superficially thought through and unwilling to address existing hegemonic technologies of socioeconomic and cultural power. Funders and administrators often fail to interrogate themselves or acknowledge that problems in implementation may be associated with their own practices. Factors that inhibit the programmes are located in the minds or communities of those being addressed. Such approaches perpetuate simplistic, top-down programme implementation at the expense of the fully exercised community participation to which programmes are discursively committed. Campbell pointed out how community participation technologies can therefore have dual effects, assisting community members to gain more control of their circumstances, but also helping those administering the programmes to assert their own control over communities. Such appropriations of participation and empowerment discourses, because they fail to interrogate the dynamics of power and inequality and the ethics of relationality involved in HIV programmes, undo democratic citizenship and promote an oligarchic version.

Following a similar argument, Wilbraham addressed questions of citizenship through transcripts of group discussions about parenting and children's sexual behaviour in relation to HIV transmission. The discussions were generated by examining an extract from *Lovelines*, a popular magazine column addressing parenting in the context of the HIV epidemic. Wilbraham's analysis showed that expert knowledge shapes HIV citizenship, especially through the classing and racing of what counts as expertise regarding sexual health and parenting. Magazine experts call on parents to inoculate their children against HIV risk, so that HIV citizenship is equated with responsibility towards others. Like Campbell, Wilbraham argued that such forms of expertise can be colonising, limiting and constraining, when they could be enabling. But also, consistent with the contested nature of HIV citizenship, Wilbraham showed how such expertise can be taken up as a form of empowerment and a means of reconfiguring parenting practices for the current circumstances of the epidemic. Wilbraham argued that HIV prevention technologies cannot therefore be understood as universal or designed to perfect the transmission of expertise. What can be done is to expand the 'critical space' (this volume, page 102) for dialogue regarding, for example, parenting and HIV, such that circulating imperatives and normativities can be variously exploited or dispensed with through reflexive practice. Wilbraham's 'critical space' is reminiscent of consciencisation and resonates with Campbell, who referred to Freire-style principles of critical literacy (this volume, page 22) to ground her formulation of effective HIV work. Several other chapters touch on similar principles of carefully worked-through accountability, dialogue and negotiation. Davis for instance argued that because the implications of ART knowledge are not solely technical but also deeply ethical, sustained, critical conversations are needed to address the implications and nuances for HIV citizenship.

These kinds of address to the imbrication of citizenship and HIV technologies will continue to be crucial for the development of transnational understandings of the pandemic and of HIV programmes.

Pragmatism

A frame of understanding with particular salience and insistence for HIV technologies is that of pragmatism. Pragmatism is commensurable with the operation and analysis of technologies, because it is concerned with what can be effected, the diverse and complicated technological assemblages that achieve such effects, and the articulations of contingent, equivalent relationships within and between them. Pragmatism is indeed required for negotiations of citizenship of the kind that appear in this book and for reaching some provisional end to the particularities explored here. In addition, pragmatism, since it is directed towards real possibilities of technologies, towards potentiation and not just the virtual, also allows us to follow specific lines of technological co-production or potentiation (West, 1989).

Pragmatism is a variant of realism anchored in the field of human action. It allows us to understand the work of highly ideologically committed HIV programmes such as Partners In Health and the Treatment Action Campaign that nevertheless manage to operate within the messy nexuses of local and international politics and socioeconomic divisions. It gives us a double vision of both the fantasised control by HIV's subjectification offered by psychosocial technologies, like those Wilbraham describes – as if there could indeed be a subject with complete safety, no risk, no HIV – and the possibilities for effective personal and collective action enabled at times by such technologies. It helps us to get a grip on the place of HIV in 'postcolonial' contexts as responses to the pandemic's reprise of colonial violence (Mbembe, 2001), and in the developed world where HIV is either secreted or expelled (Patton, 2002). At the same time it lets us use an antagonistic relation to these repetitions and exclusions to construct a provisional and revisable future (Mouffe, 2005) towards which HIV technologies can work.

The final theme we would thus like to address concerns pragmatics: the importance of situated, reflexive practices for effective HIV technologies. Pragmatism expresses themes already discussed: it encompasses the potentiating effects of HIV technologies, articulated together; questions over the ontological status of watersheds and dichotomies in HIV narratives; and tensions within HIV citizenship to do with volition and requirement, related concerns of ethical relationality, and diverse levels and directions of power. Several authors in this volume asserted the need to acknowledge the practical, everyday efforts of affected communities and the agencies that assist them, making reference to such notions as 'pragmatic citizenship' (Abdullah and Squire), 'situated dialogues' (Campbell, Wilbraham and Davis) and 'phronesis' (Mykhalovskiy). These authors also identified a necessary move away from the political and the rhetorical towards what could be called a focus on 'administrative governmentality' in HIV analyses (Abdullah and Squire). Campbell showed how the language of 'community participation' can become a mandate for decidedly disempowering forms of administrative practice. Likewise, Mykhalovskiy noted how the discourse of treatment and prevention integration may not support the good health of people with HIV or of the public in general. These arguments serve to draw attention to the necessarily critical dimensions of the pragmatic uses of HIV technologies.

Abdullah and Squire advocated for an acknowledgement of the technologies of partnership that have helped make the ART roll-out in the Western Cape an exemplar. They referenced specific practices that helped the roll-out, including ART's devolvement to primary health care environments, and the integration of locally decided education for ART, healthy lives and safer sex. The point of their argument is not that these formulations will work everywhere. The Western Cape roll-out has wider relevance since its principal feature was to acknowledge local enabling and constraining factors in everyday practices. This pragmatism is important in that it allows consistent attention to the particularities of HIV technologies, something that also enables the potentiations deriving from spatiotemporal relationships between technologies. Pragmatism extends to citizenship technologies: as Abdullah and Squire described, the Western Cape roll-out relied on a presiding understanding of equivalence co-existing with antagonism. The HIV affected and non-affected can join in action on the basis of their commonalities, without erasing particularities. This form of citizenship can help mobilise individuals and communities under a guarantee of equivalence that does not depend on sameness. It is an approach consistent with the elements Campbell specifies as comprising 'AIDS competent communities', in particular, shared purpose, solidarity and effective partnerships between communities of interest and national and international agencies of HIV governance.

Mykhalovskiy suggested something similar when arguing the salience of phronesis – practical wisdom – for thinking about the integration of HIV treatment and prevention. Mykhalovskiy argued that the most tenable method of integrating treatment and prevention depends on proper community engagement and the acknowledgment of the expertise and capacities of communities that are in the best position to address client needs. At the same time, Mykhalovskiy described accommodation, the reconfiguration of responsibility and the future-oriented directions of the technologies with which he is concerned. Similarly, Flowers and Davis argued that approaches to ART and its implications for HIV prevention need to take account of the lived experience of those affected by HIV and the ethical implications that arise. Flowers's chapter worked consistently with the pragmatics of 'experience', with phenomena like stigmatisation that, despite apparently sufficient explanations and interventions, resist and persist. Davis's finishing emphasis on technologies of hope again returned us to pragmatism's critical, tangential relation to metaphysics. By stepping outside conventional epistemological categories, pragmatism – and this chapter – takes a stepwise and revisible path, rather than a faith-infused leap, towards a future for which hope is a strategy, not a teleology or method of subjectification.

Conclusion

The case studies presented in this book help establish means for addressing the ART possibility era in ways that resist crude determinisms and globalisations. The book's method has been to seek out nuance and particularity where there has typically been simplification and dualism. The analyses have been diverse, including meta-analyses of prevention evaluation science, institutional ethnographies, focus groups and interviews with those affected by the epidemic, and accounts of HIV technologies informed by cultural studies and science and technology studies. Chapter writers have creatively undermined or reversed orthodox accounts of the epidemic after ART and related technological turnings in its governance, to establish new modes of analysis. They have explored alterities and counter-discourses, hitherto submerged or ignored, to elaborate on the conditions of possibility for HIV subjects. The writers have brought the psychosocial features of HIV back into relationship with an ascendant biotechnological rationalisation of pandemic governance, to reveal the problematic aspects of some HIV technologies. Writers have offered new insights concerning the persisting difficulties of the post-ART era, such as the putative effects of ART on HIV prevention and vice versa. One of the richest dimensions of this volume is how each chapter has variously revealed ethical, political and cultural in connection with technical and administrative technologies of the treatment possibility era. The writers have not ignored how ART and other HIV technologies can and do have life-changing effects for individuals, those who care for them, communities and nations. Nor have they underestimated the value of HIV prevention for people with HIV and those affected by the epidemic, including the capacities that ART and other biomedical interventions may have in this respect. In this conclusion, we have referenced notions of potentiation, citizenship and pragmatics intersecting with transnational and intra-national particularities, as a way of suggesting how the volume has sustained a double engagement with continuity and disjunction. It is our argument that such forms of analysis are important for articulating ways of thinking and acting in current and future configurations of HIV technologies.

References

Butler, J. (2005) *Giving an account of oneself* (Fordham, NY: Fordham University Press).

Campbell, C. (2003) *Letting them die?* (Oxford: James Currey).

Davis, M. (2007) 'Identity, expertise and HIV risk in a case study of reflexivity and medical technologies', *Sociology*, 41, 6, 1003–19.

Deleuze, G. and Parnet, C. (1977) *Dialogues* (New York: Columbia University Press).

Dilley, J., Woods, W. and McFarland, W. (1997), 'Are advances in treatment changing views about high-risk sex?' *The New England Journal of Medicine*, 337, 7, 501–2.

Elford, J. (2006), 'Changing patterns of sexual behaviour in the era of highly active antiretroviral therapy', *Current Opinion in Infectious Diseases*, 19, 26–32.

Farmer, P. (2001) *Infections and inequalities* (Los Angeles, CA: University of California Press).

Fleet, R. (2009) 'Bare faced cheek' *Positive Nation*, 142 http://www.positivenation.co.uk/regulars/index.php, accessed 09.06.09.

Flowers, P., Davis, M., Hart, G., Imrie, J., Rosengarten, M. and Frankis, J. (2006), 'Diagnosis and stigma and identity amongst HIV positive Black Africans living in the UK', *Psychology and Health*, 21, 1, 109–22.

Foucault, M. (1980) *History of sexuality volume 1* (London: Allen Lane).
Kelly, J., Hoffman, R., Rompa, D. and Gray, M. (1998), 'Protease inhibitor combination therapies and perceptions of gay men regarding AIDS severity and the need to maintain safer sex', *AIDS*, 12, F91–F95.
Laclau, E. and Mouffe, C. (1985) *Hegemony and socialist strategy*. (London: Verso).
—— (2001) [1985] *Hegemony and socialist strategy* (London: Verso).
Lana, B. (2009) *From risk to reason: understanding young people's perception of HIV risk in South Africa*. Ph.D. thesis, University of York.
Magona, S. (2008) *Beauty's gift* (Cape Town: Kwela Books).
Mazibuko, L. (2008) 'Address the people's needs', *Sowetan*, 5 November, http://www.sowetan.co.za/Columnists/LuckyMazibuko/Article.aspx?id=877700, accessed 09.06.09.
Mbembe, A. (2001) *On the postcolony* (Los Angeles, CA: University of California Press).
Monk, D. (2009) 'Reckless trials? Contextualising the criminalisation of the sexual transmission of HIV', *Radical Philosophy*, 156, July/August. http://www.radicalphilosophy.com/default.asp?channel_id=2187&editorial_id=28201, accessed 1 October 2009.
Mouffe, C. (1992) 'Democratic citizenship and the political community', in *Dimensions of radical democracy: pluralism, citizenship and community*, C. Mouffe (ed.) (London: Verso).
—— (2005) *On the political* (London: Routledge).
Patton, C. (2002) *Globalizing AIDS* (Minneapolis, MN: University of Minnesota Press).
Rabinow, P. (1999) *French DNA: Trouble in purgatory* (Chicago: University of Chicago Press).
—— (2004) 'Assembling ethics in an ecology of ignorance', First conference on synthetic biology, MIT, 10–12 June, http://openwetware.org/images/7/7a/SB1.0_Rabinow.pdf, accessed 09.06.09.
—— (2007) *Marking time: On the anthropology of the contemporary* (Princeton, NJ: Princeton University Press).
Remien, R., O'Leary, A., Halkitis, P. and Hays, R. (1998), 'Perceptions, attitudes and sexual risk among HIV-positive men with undetectable plasma viral loads', *Poster presented at the 12th World AIDS Conference, Geneva, 28 June–3 July*.
Steinberg, J. (2008) *Sizwe's test* (New York: Simon and Shuster).
West, C. (1989) *The American evasion of philosophy* (Madison, WI: University of Wisconsin Press).

Index